Understanding Childhood Obesity

Understanding Health and Sickness Series
Miriam Bloom, Ph.D.
General Editor

Understanding Childhood Obesity

J. Clinton Smith, M.D., M.P.H.

University Press of Mississippi
Jackson

Copyright © 1999 by the University Press of Mississippi
Manufactured in the United States of America

02 01 00 99   4 3 2 1

The paper in this book meets the guidelines for permanence and durability
of the Committee on Production Guidelines for Book Longevity of the
Council on Library Resources.

Illustrations by Regan Causey Tuder

Library of Congress Cataloging-in-Publication Data

Smith, J. Clinton, 1939–
    Understanding childhood obesity / J. Clinton Smith.
        p.   cm.—(Understanding health and sickness series)
    Includes bibliographical references and index.
        ISBN 1-57806-133-4 (cloth : alk. paper).—ISBN 1-57806-134-2
    (pbk. : alk. paper)
        1. Obesity in children—Prevention.   2. Obesity in children—
    Psychological aspects.   3. Children—Nutrition.   4. Behavior
    therapy for children.   I. Title.   II. Series.
    RJ399.C6S63   1999
    618.92'398—dc21   98-44680
                                                        CIP

British Library Cataloging-in-Publication Data available

Contents

Acknowledgments

I am grateful to Jim Joransen, David Braden, Makram Ebeid, and Charlie Gaymes, my colleagues in the Division of Cardiology of the Department of Pediatrics at the University of Mississippi Medical Center, for allowing me time to write this book. Only through their support has the Pediatric Preventive Cardiology Clinic become a reality. I am also appreciative of the physicians, nurses, and dietitians who have made referrals to our clinics. Without the support of the Mississippi State Department of Health, our clinics could not have met in various communities across the state, and families would have been unable to obtain assistance.

I would also like to thank the editor of the Understanding Health and Sickness Series, Dr. Miriam Bloom, for her patient efforts. In spite of her many other activities in the community and around the state, she always found time to scrutinize drafts of this book. Her suggestions were consistently on target, and she helped me translate the scientific jargon into everyday language (I take full responsibility for any lapses in this regard).

Two other individuals were extremely helpful in the book's preparation. Dr. Richard Troiano of the National Center for Health Statistics graciously provided me with unpublished data from the National Health and Nutrition Examination Survey III concerning overweight and obesity among children. Dr. Harold White, Emeritus Professor of Biochemistry at the University of Mississippi Medical Center, reviewed the material on digestion and energy and made invaluable comments and suggestions.

Most of all, I am indebted to Lois, my wife of thirty years, for her unconditional love and her even temperament. She always makes it easy for me to do what I need to do.

Introduction

Hardly a week goes by that a magazine or tabloid newspaper doesn't feature an article about someone who is overweight, who is trying to lose weight, or who should be trying to lose weight. "How-to" books about weight loss are available in great number. We know about celebrities such as Oprah Winfrey, Elizabeth Taylor, David Letterman, and Tommy Lasorda who have successfully dealt with their own weight problems. Others, including swimmer Lynne Cox, musicians Kate Smith, Fats Domino, and Chubby Checker, singer Cass Elliot, Chicago Bear "Refrigerator" Perry, and most professional football linemen, have used excess weight to their advantage. Thanks to overweight opera singers, "It's not over 'til the fat lady sings" is a national aphorism. Americans seem obsessed with weight loss. We talk about how much weight we want to lose or how much we have lost as frequently as we talk about the weather. Our weight and what we're trying to do about it is always a timely subject. And our conversations about weight usually have something to do with our appearance—the way we look to other people.

Self-image is unquestionably important. But there is a far more serious aspect of being overweight that we don't talk about much, and that is how this condition can affect our health and longevity. Consider the following facts:

First, about 500,000 Americans die each year from diseases of the heart, especially coronary artery disease, or disease of the blood vessels supplying blood to the heart. This disease doesn't just develop overnight. It is a slow, degenerative process that can begin in childhood. Adults who are obese, who have high blood pressure or abnormal blood cholesterol levels, who use tobacco, and who engage in little or no physical activity appear to be at high risk for this degenerative process (Eckel et al. 1998). Yet mounting evidence indicates that if children who have risk factors can be identified and appropriate corrective action taken, there might be less chance that they will have heart disease when they become adults (Bao et al. 1997).

Second, in the years 1988–94, about 35 percent of American adults over 20 years of age (nearly 60 million people) were obese, up from 25 percent in the years 1976–80. The news concerning children was also startling: the proportion of overweight children (6- to 11-year-olds) climbed from 20 percent in the period 1976–80 to 27 percent between 1988 and 1994; the proportion of overweight adolescents (12- to 17-year-olds) rose from 16 percent to 27 percent over the same time. Approximately 5 million children and adolescents are now classified as being obese. Many, but not all, obese youngsters become obese adults, and many obese adults can trace their excess weight to faulty nutrition and physical activity patterns established during childhood.

A glaring incongruity exists in Americans' ideas of health care. On the one hand, we have great expectations: we know that when we become ill or injured, we will receive the very best care available in the world, and that our doctors and hospitals will be paid by our insurance programs. If we survive a heart attack, we go to state-of-the-art coronary care units, have coronary artery bypass grafts, take drugs that help keep coronary arteries open, and receive rehabilitation services for damaged hearts. Astonishing, but costly, technological advances in health care since 1950 have made such interventions possible, and we have welcomed them and now take them for granted.

The incongruity is that we don't seem to realize that it is within our power as human beings to prevent, or at least delay, some diseases. Many heart attacks, strokes, cancers, and other diseases and conditions would not occur if we were effective in preventing obesity.

My purpose in writing this book is to suggest that childhood is the best time to prevent obesity and its later consequences. The book is intended to assist families, teachers, health providers, and other friends of children in understanding better why some children become obese, how being obese can result in health problems in childhood and in adulthood, and what can be done to help youngsters become healthy adults. I have drawn on the wisdom and contributions of professionals in many different fields who are serious students of the problem of obesity, including basic science researchers, dietitians, exercise physiologists, psychologists, and physicians. I hope that readers will use the book to expand their knowledge of this critical public health issue.

I begin with a discussion of the major ways in which obesity is an important health problem and why we need to do something at both the individual and the population levels. The first chapter also explains some of the consequences of obesity in children and in adults.

In the second chapter I explain the process of classifying a child's weight and height as "normal" or "abnormal," how a diagnosis of obesity is made in children, and what the difficulties are in comparing different populations of children. I also identify groups of children and adolescents who are most likely to become obese adults.

Chapters 3, 4, and 5 are concerned with how energy is taken into the body and used and with how energy imbalance leads to obesity. In chapter 3 I review how food is broken down into molecules in the digestive tract and how these molecules are absorbed into the bloodstream, enter the cells of the body, and are then either used as immediate energy sources or stored for future energy needs. In chapter 4, I explain how energy from food is supplied and used. I also introduce the energy balance equation, which is the basis for measuring energy intake and expenditure. Some of the possible reasons for obesity in childhood are presented in chapter 5, including evidence from both behavioral and metabolic research. The chapter focuses on the importance of genetic and environmental factors associated with obesity.

Chapter 6 examines the question "Can obesity be prevented in American children?" I try to emphasize the difference between *hoping* that prevention can take place because of successful demonstration projects and *realistic expectations* within the context of the powerful environmental influences affecting children's daily eating and exercise habits. I cite examples of the ways in which parents, government, schools, and health professionals have attempted to prevent obesity, and comment on the likelihood that prevention efforts will be expanded.

Techniques used in treatment of obese children are discussed in chapter 7. Several approaches are defined, and the traditional elements of treatment, such as nutrition education, decreased calorie and fat intake, increased physical activity, and behavior modification are detailed. Examples of aggressive medical and surgical management, including a discussion of drugs to treat obesity, are presented. I also introduce the reader to the "continuous care and problem solving model" of treatment, and explain how this works in our pediatric treatment clinics at the University of Mississippi Medical Center.

Finally, chapter 8 contains a summary of exciting new developments that have taken place in obesity research in recent years, including the discovery of leptin and the leptin receptor and the promising genetics research that may finally explain why obesity develops in some individuals but not in others.

I have cited references only to sources other than material that can be found in standard textbooks of basic science and clinical medicine.

For me, the richest source of information has been the hundreds of obese children and their families in Mississippi who have sought assistance in our clinics. In getting to know them, learning about their family and school environments, and identifying with their struggles to change their eating and physical activity patterns, I have come to realize how little is known about the origins and treatment of obesity in childhood. Without knowing those children, I would have had little incentive to write this book. They continue to be superb teachers.

Understanding Childhood Obesity

1. Why Is Obesity an Important Health Problem in America?

Leave gormandizing. Know the grave doth gape
For thee thrice wider than for other men.

William Shakespeare,
Henry IV, Part II (quoted in Bray 1985)

Twentieth-century Americans have enjoyed a standard of living unparalleled in history. We are well nourished, we live in attractive and affordable houses, we have clean water and milk and good sewage systems, and we are largely free from the scourges suffered by so much of the rest of the world, such as malaria, yellow fever, rheumatic fever, blindness due to parasites, and malnutrition. We are a well-educated nation. Many of us work 40-hour weeks, have guaranteed vacations, and are free to enjoy the fruits of our labor before we grow too old. Our health care system has provided us with powerful drugs and technologies that cure illnesses and prolong lives.

Yet we are not entirely well. The health problems dominating the early part of this century have been replaced by a new morbidity—diseases brought on by our living habits. Like other industrialized countries, we now have high rates of heart disease, cancer, strokes, and obesity. Nearly 60 million American adults between the ages of 20 and 75 years—1 in 3—are obese. One of every 4 U. S. adults smokes cigarettes regularly, a habit usually acquired in adolescence and linked to several fatal conditions. Since most of us are now city dwellers, we can't conveniently walk to work or to visit our neighbors. And, thanks to labor-saving technologies, we have discovered how to work without sweating.

We reward ourselves at the end of the day with big meals and evenings of watching television. We are sports enthusiasts and spectators, but frequently avoid physical activity ourselves. A fourth of adult Americans have high blood pressure or high blood cholesterol. Many don't realize it because they haven't taken the time to find out, while others know but are unwilling or unable to take available medications.

The fact is that many Americans want to have good health but don't want to pay the personal price to achieve it. We undertake to live what we see as "the good life," and, if something goes wrong, we rely on our doctors and hospitals and technology and drugs to fix us up and get us going again. And since we don't want to worry about the expense, we say "just bill my insurance company." Those of us in the health professions do a pretty good job of treating disease, but we're not always doing so well at getting the message out that a lot of death and disability can be prevented. Government and health insurance companies give lip service to the idea of prevention, but education in this area is infrequently compensated, and it has not been a high priority among health practitioners. Managed health care may eventually modify this deficiency.

Many of us have not yet connected obesity to possible poor health. Obesity is a chronic condition—not an acute, urgent, and headline-grabbing disease like AIDS or meningitis—and is therefore likely to receive less attention. Its effects are insidious, its origins are complex and poorly understood, and its treatment is often discouraging. But obesity can be prevented if the American people will that it be so (National Institutes of Health 1985; Lew 1985; Pi-Sunyer 1991; Dietz et al. 1993; Alpert et al. 1993).

This chapter explores a number of ways in which obesity is a major health problem among Americans. Some of the complications of obesity, such as heart disease, begin in childhood, but do not become apparent until adulthood. If we are to understand why some adults are healthy and others are not, we must first understand how habits that we acquire early in life can affect our health later.

Obesity and Overall Mortality

Obese people do not live as long as other people. Life insurance company studies done early in the 20th century showed that, as the weight of individuals increases above an optimal level, the probability of dying increases, too. In 1979 the American Cancer Society confirmed that finding in a 12-year study of 750,000 people which took into consideration their state of health and whether they smoked. The study also found that men and women who were 5-15 percent *below* average weight were likely to live longest. The most common causes of death among men in the American Cancer Society study were diseased coronary arteries, stroke, and digestive diseases. The same was true in women, except that diabetes was also common. Obese men and women were also more likely to die of cancer than were those who were not obese.

Let's find out why obesity is an important health problem among Americans. Which organs or systems can it affect, and what happens then?

Effect of Obesity on the Heart and Blood Vessels

Obesity is strongly associated with diseases of the heart and blood vessels in several ways. First, obese people appear to be more likely to develop disease of the coronary arteries, which are the vessels that supply the heart muscle with blood. Blood flow in those arteries can be blocked due to a complex process called *atherosclerosis*, which is more common in obese than in nonobese adults. Blockage of coronary arteries can cause part of the heart muscle to die (a *myocardial infarction*, or *heart attack*).

After a heart attack, the heart may not be able to pump adequate amounts of blood to other vital organs, such as the brain, lungs, and kidneys, and death or disability may result.

Second, obesity also can directly affect the heart muscle, independent of its effect on the coronary arteries. This condition is called *obesity cardiomyopathy*. Third, heart disease can occur when obesity causes *abnormal functioning of the lungs*. Finally, obese people are very likely to have *high blood pressure* (*hypertension*), which can damage both the coronary arteries and the heart muscle.

Since coronary artery disease is responsible for the deaths of about 500,000 people in the United States annually (roughly 25 percent of the 2 million or so Americans dying each year) and causes 1.4 million nonfatal heart attacks each year, let's begin with a discussion of this condition.

Many studies have shown that coronary artery disease occurs more often in people having high blood pressure and abnormal blood cholesterol levels, who exercise little or not at all, who smoke cigarettes, who have diabetes, and who are obese. One way in which obesity seems to lead to coronary artery disease is first to cause some of the other problems just mentioned, such as abnormal blood cholesterol levels or high blood pressure. In this sense, obesity is an *indirect* cause of coronary artery disease, meaning that its effects on the heart and blood vessels take place because other abnormal conditions have already developed.

But obesity also appears to have an effect on the heart and blood vessels that does not depend on the development of intermediate conditions (Higgins et al. 1987). For example, excess body fat can be stored either viscerally (in the abdomen, surrounding the liver and intestines) or peripherally (in the upper arms, the thighs, and the buttocks). Although the amount of visceral fat is more difficult to measure than peripheral fat, studies have shown that the association of visceral fat with coronary artery disease is independent of other risk factors, such as high blood pressure or diabetes. Why excess visceral fat is so much more strongly associated with coronary artery disease than excess peripheral fat is not well understood.

Does coronary artery disease ever occur in children? Only rarely. However, the process begins in early childhood; it is now well established that deposits of fat and fibrous tissue are present in the blood vessels of children as young as 4 or 5 years old. While a heart attack caused by this process would be unusual in a child or adolescent, it would not be in a 30- or 40-year-old. The important thing is that, even though the process of atherosclerosis may be inevitable, the rate at which it occurs probably can be slowed down, and the death and disability that it causes can be delayed.

Another Way in Which Obesity Can Affect the Heart

Body fat is a living tissue. It doesn't just sit there and do nothing! It has to obtain oxygen and to get rid of waste material, and therefore has to have a blood supply. As we put on extra fat, we develop extra blood vessels, red blood cells, and plasma to carry oxygen and nutrition to it. The amount of blood in our circulatory system increases, and, since the heart has to pump all the blood that comes into it, the two pumping chambers of the heart (ventricles) may dilate to handle the extra volume, with their walls becoming thicker (hypertrophic) to pump the blood out with extra force (fig. 1.1). *Hypertrophy* of the heart muscle means that extra muscle tissue is added to the heart, in the same way that weight lifters put on extra muscle tissue. Excessive dilation and hypertrophy can eventually weaken the ability of the heart to pump blood. And if the heart eventually fails to pump out all the blood that comes to it, heart failure occurs. Heart failure due to obesity is called obesity cardiomyopathy.

Can obesity-related heart failure occur in children? Yes, but it happens only rarely, and mainly in children who are extremely obese. But even in children who are only moderately obese,

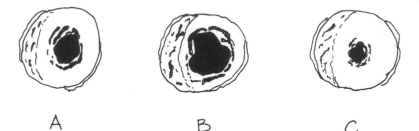

A   B   C

FIG. I.I. Cross section of the left ventricle of the heart, comparing dilation and hypertrophy with the normal state. (A) Normal cavity size and wall thickness. (B) Dilation of the ventricular cavity, with thinning of the ventricular wall. (C) Hypertrophy (thickening) of the ventricular wall, with normal or decreased ventricular cavity size.

increased blood volume can affect the size of the heart chambers and the thickness of their walls.

Effect of Obesity on the Respiratory System

One of the most common consequences of obesity in children and adults is *obstructive sleep apnea,* caused by excessive fatty tissue in the back of the throat blocking air flow from the nose to the lungs during sleep. Relaxation of the throat and neck muscles during sleep allows excess fat in the walls of the throat to protrude into the airway, causing partial or total obstruction of air flow to the lungs. Loud snoring may be the only sign of partial obstruction. But if the airway becomes totally obstructed, normal breathing may be interrupted for as long as 30 or more seconds. This causes the person to awaken and change positions to overcome the obstruction. The quality of sleep and rest is poor, causing daytime sleepiness, which can, of course, result in a poor attention span and poor school or work performance. Sleep apnea may be life threatening in many children and adults, and surgery to remove the obstructive tissue is often required. In addition, chronic airway obstruction from any cause, including excessively large adenoids, often causes *hypoxemia,* a condition in which the oxygen in the circulatory system is low. This can eventually result in high pressure in the blood vessels that carry blood to the lungs, and cause thickening (hypertrophy) of the walls of the right ventricle. Heart failure can result.

A condition closely related to obstructive sleep apnea is frequently seen in severely obese people and is called the *Pickwickian syndrome*, after Joe the fat boy in Charles Dickens's novel *The Pickwick Papers*. Its technical name is *obesity hypoventilation syndrome*, which simply means that, because of obesity, not as much air enters the lungs as ordinarily would. This can happen when the amount of fat stored in the abdomen and chest is so great that the chest and diaphragm cannot move in a normal manner. It's like wearing a very tight girdle or waistband around the chest and abdomen. The affected individual has to work much harder to breathe, and needs more oxygen for this extra work. However, less oxygen is available since the lungs cannot expand normally. In addition, when any part of the lung does not fully expand, the blood cannot get its full supply of oxygen. The net effect is hypoxemia. As in obstructive sleep apnea, sleep quality may be poor and daytime sleepiness is common. Usually, low blood oxygen levels stimulate the breathing centers in the brain to speed up the breathing rate. But over time, the brain centers can become less responsive to low oxygen levels, and hypoxemia worsens. Chronic hypoxemia due to the obesity hypoventilation syndrome can result in heart failure by the same mechanisms as those found in obstructive sleep apnea. Both these conditions, of course, can occur in the same individual.

Obesity and High Blood Pressure

Obese people, regardless of age, are more likely to develop high blood pressure (hypertension) than nonobese people. American adults (defined as 20–75 years old) who are obese are 3 times more likely than nonobese adults to develop this condition. Even those whose blood pressure is not high enough to treat with medication often have "high normal" pressures. Why obesity is associated with hypertension is not completely understood, but it probably has something to do with increased blood volume (discussed above) and increased resistance of blood vessels to blood flow. In any case, untreated hypertension places a strain on the left side of the heart, causing it to become hypertrophic. In time, the heart can fail. Untreated hypertension also can cause narrowing and obstruction of the blood vessels supplying the heart, resulting in heart attacks.

Remember that hypertension can begin in childhood. Although many obese children have hypertension, it rarely causes heart failure or stroke at that stage of life. But if high blood pressure persists into adulthood and is not treated, the consequences can be serious.

Effect of Obesity on Blood Lipids

Lipid is the scientific term for a substance that is soluble (can be dissolved) in fat. Lipids are essential to life; they perform many valuable roles in maintaining good health. Lipids come from our diets, or can be manufactured by the liver from dietary carbohydrates (starches, sugars). Other lipids that we obtain from the food we eat and make in our bodies are known as *sterols*. Cholesterol is the most important example of a sterol in humans. The two kinds of lipids that are most important to the health of obese people are cholesterol and triglycerides (defined in chapter 3).

We can be born with abnormal levels of certain blood lipids, which can cause atherosclerosis. On the other hand, some people can acquire abnormal blood lipid levels if they become obese, smoke cigarettes, are sedentary, or have excessive dietary fat intake. The risk of having abnormal blood cholesterol levels is about 1½ times higher in obese than in nonobese adults. The first

line of treatment in obese children or adults with abnormal lipid
levels is weight loss.

Obesity and Type II (Adult-onset, Non-insulin-dependent) Diabetes

In the United States, about 15.7 million people, or 5.9 percent
of the population, have diabetes, a disease characterized by
abnormally high blood sugar (*glucose*) levels. One-third of these
are undiagnosed. Type II diabetes is the form that commonly
occurs in adulthood, as opposed to type I (juvenile) diabetes,
which has its onset in childhood and currently affects about
120,000 children under the age of 20 years. Type II diabetes
accounts for 90–95 percent of all diagnosed diabetes, and can
usually be controlled by diet, exercise, oral medications, and, in
some cases, insulin (National Institute of Diabetes and Digestive
and Kidney Diseases Home Page 1997). Diabetes has ranked
among the 10 leading causes of death among Americans since
1932 and currently results in about 36,000 deaths annually. The
risk of diabetes increases with both age and obesity: people
who are 50 percent above their optimal weight are 5 times as
likely to be diabetic. Of great concern is a recent report that
adult-onset diabetes is being found with increasing frequency
in obese adolescents (Pinhas-Hamiel et al. 1996). People with
either type I or type II diabetes are likely to develop coronary
artery disease, abnormal blood lipid levels, high blood pressure,
strokes, blindness, gangrene of their feet or legs, and kidney
failure. Children born to diabetic mothers are more likely to
have birth defects and die during infancy.

Our discussion thus far has concentrated on the life-
threatening conditions that are frequently found among obese
individuals. Other consequences of obesity, which are not
necessarily as drastic, nevertheless can result in chronic illness
and disability.

Psychosocial Consequences of Obesity

Although many obese children and adults seem to be perfectly happy with their weights, others may have poor images of themselves and become socially withdrawn. Some experience serious depression and may require psychotherapy or medication. Parents know the heartbreak of having their obese children teased by other children, or being told (often by adults) that they don't have the self-discipline to lose weight, or that their families don't care enough about them and their health to correct the problem. Youngsters who are obese and want to lose weight often give "being able to do the things that other kids are doing" as their reason; they want to go where their peers are going, wear the same kinds of clothes, be invited out on dates, and form the normal everyday relationships that their friends have. If they do not develop those relationships, some may grow up lacking social skills, and they may have difficulty in being accepted by colleges, in finding and keeping a job, and in forming the intimacy and trust necessary for marriage. The negative attitudes of nonobese children toward those who are obese or otherwise "different" are formed early in life. In one survey, children as young as 6 years of age rated obese children as "less likable" than those who aren't, and rated obese kids even more negatively than children having facial disfigurement or missing limbs.

Obese children or adults may overeat, feel bad about doing so, but then eat again to feel better. This is referred to as *binge eating*. On the other hand, obese girls and young women often become preoccupied with their weight and may go to the opposite extreme, refusing to eat or eating only very small amounts of food, a condition known as *anorexia*, or forcing themselves to regurgitate after eating, which is called *bulimia*. Anorexia and bulimia can be resistant to treatment, and can result in death from starvation.

Many obese young people as well as adults seem perfectly happy with themselves, appearing to be confident, sociable, and well liked by their peers. They have accepted their obesity as a fact of life. They may be just as talented, well educated, and socially mature as anyone else. Organizations such as the National Association to Advance Fat Acceptance enable obese individuals to communicate with each other and share ideas. *Radiance* is a magazine for large women. In addition, various cultural and social groups may have different perceptions of what constitutes the ideal body image. For example, African American families, especially the grandparents, may often perceive obesity to be a sign of robustness and leanness an indication of disease or poor health.

Effects of Obesity on Other Body Systems

Obese children are likely to develop *tibia vara deformity*, also known as *tibia vara*, or *Blount's disease*, a condition in which the growth plate of the tibia (the larger bone in the lower leg) develops abnormally. This can result in severe bowing of the legs, which limits a person's ability to run, jump, or even walk. A second problem frequently seen in obese children is *slipped capital femoral epiphysis*. In this rare but extremely serious condition, the growth plate of the head of the femur (the single large bone of the upper leg which joins the pelvis bone) becomes detached from the main body of the femur, causing pain and inability to walk. This condition can interfere with the blood supply to the hip, causing severe damage to the hip joint, and can result in permanent disability. About 75 percent of children with either of the above conditions are obese.

Obese adults are particularly prone to develop *osteoarthritis*, which is a painful swelling of some of the joints and which may limit movement, as well as to sometimes-disabling low back pain.

Obese children are frequently taller than their peers and appear to be larger than normal, not only because of excessive body fat, but also because they have more lean body mass (more muscle tissue and bigger bones). Obese girls may experience early onset of menstruation, and are likely to develop secondary sexual characteristics, such as breast development and the appearance of pubic and other body hair, earlier than their normal-weight counterparts. On the other hand, they are more likely to have menstrual periods which are irregular in occurrence and length and to have masculine characteristics such as coarse skin and facial hair. They may be less fertile than normal as they mature, a condition frequently referred to as *polycystic ovary disease*,[1] which can be both a consequence and a cause of obesity.

Obese males frequently have decreased sperm production, as well as lower levels of testosterone, the primary male hormone. Many obese males have been found to have increased levels of some female hormones, which may cause excessive breast size.

Some children and adults develop fatty livers, a condition referred to as *hepatic steatosis*, which is associated with abnormally high liver function tests. The long-term effects of this condition in children are not well understood, but concern has been expressed that some cases of fatty liver can be associated with cirrhosis in later life.

Gallstones occur 3 or 4 times more frequently in obese than in nonobese persons, especially those who are attempting to lose weight. Children as well as adults can be affected.

Some obese adults (especially women), as well as a few obese children, develop chronic headaches because of increased pressure around the brain and spinal cord. This symptom is similar to one occurring in people with brain tumors. The condition is referred to as *pseudotumor cerebri*, meaning that symptoms are *similar to* those accompanying brain tumors, but do not occur *because of* brain tumors. The condition usually resolves with weight loss.

Obese women appear to have higher rates of uterine, cervical, ovarian, breast, and gallbladder cancers (Huang et al. 1997; · Ballard-Barbash et al. 1996). The reported association between obesity and cancer of the colon and rectum is unclear (Shike 1996). Cancer associated with obesity has not been reported in childhood.

Costs of Diseases Associated with Obesity in the United States

Nearly 80 percent of patients with type II diabetes are obese, and much of the estimated $19 billion direct costs of health care due to this disease is attributable to obesity.

Nearly 70 percent of diagnosed cases of diseases of the heart and blood vessels are related to obesity; obesity accounts for $22.2 billion spent annually on heart disease, or 19 percent of the total cost of diagnosis and treatment.

The annual cost of diagnosing and treating high blood pressure is about $1.5 billion. High blood pressure affects about one-fourth of American adults, and obesity doubles a person's chances of having this condition.

About $2.4 billion, or 30 percent of the total amount spent annually on gallbladder disease and surgery, is related to obesity.

Americans spend about $33 billion annually, including money for diets and exercise products, in their efforts to lose weight. Little wonder that we call it the weight loss "industry" (National Institute of Diabetes and Digestive and Kidney Diseases Home Page 1997).

If obesity had been prevented, the United States could have saved about $45.8 billion in 1990, or 6.8 percent of health care expenditures that year. Moreover, employers would have saved about $4 billion in 1990 if the 52.9 million days of lost productivity had not occurred (Wolf et al. 1994).

Summary

I have reviewed some of the ways in which obesity can negatively affect a person's health and productivity. If, as you read, you experienced anxiety about possible complications of obesity in yourself or in your child, that is understandable, since these difficulties are not pleasant to think about. Remember that not every obese child or adult experiences all the possible consequences. My hope is that this information will stimulate you to examine carefully how daily living habits may affect your and your family's health. The best time to undertake the prevention of obesity and its consequences is while children are young.

2. Who Is Obese, and How Do We Know?

A rose is a rose is a rose is a rose.

Gertrude Stein

We learned in the last chapter that obesity can have serious unwanted effects on a person's physical and mental health. This chapter attempts to answer the following questions: How is obesity defined, and how do we decide who is and who isn't obese? What proportion of American adults and children are obese? Has this proportion changed any over the past few years? Are obese children more likely than nonobese children to become obese adults? Were obese adults also obese when they were children? (These last two questions are not exactly the same.) Are people who share certain characteristics such as age, sex, race, or economic status more likely than others to become obese, and why is it important to know this?

Let's begin by defining the term *percentile*, which most of us see occasionally but may not understand. A percentile is a number that divides a range of numbers (a dataset) so that a given percentage lies below this number. We can take height as an example. Suppose we carefully measure the heights of a thousand 10-year-old boys. We find that the shortest boy is 48 inches (4 feet) tall, and the tallest is 60 inches (5 feet) tall. A boy's height is at the 50th percentile if 50 percent of the thousand boys have heights that are less than his. Another boy's height is at the 10th percentile if 10 percent of all the boys' heights are less than his. In the case of height and weight, we can use graphs that display percentiles for boys and girls from birth to 18 years of age, which makes correct calculation of an individual's height and weight percentile very easy (fig. 2.1).

Scientists and physicians often arbitrarily refer to measurements greater than the 95th percentile or less than the 5th percentile as being outside the range of "normal." This applies not only to body measurements, but also to laboratory tests, metabolic rates, caloric intake, and many other measurements which may relate to obesity. But we could set the "cut point" for whatever we are measuring at the 85th, 75th, or whatever percentile we wish, as long as we clearly explain to others exactly what we are doing. A child having a weight, height, or other characteristic above the 95th or below the 5th percentile does not mean that he or she is "abnormal"; it simply means that the child is at the highest or lowest end of the range of what is being measured. Indeed, no matter what is being measured, there will usually be people in the 5th percentile (5 percent have lower values) and the 95th percentile (95 percent have lower values). The work of the physician or scientist is to decide whether persons having such measurements are at greater risk for a disease or condition than are those whose measurements are between the 5th and the 95th percentiles. By understanding percentiles, we can more easily comprehend the significance of the numbers related to obesity. We will learn more about percentiles when we examine how the percentages of obesity among American adults and children have been increasing in recent years.

How do we define "obesity"? The most obvious answer is "excessive body fat." But the question actually involves several answers more complex than that, since we would have to have a good way to measure body fat in people who don't look like they have too much of it. The ideal method of defining obesity from a medical perspective would be to match a child's or young adult's weight with undesirable outcomes—such as heart attacks—experienced by the person later on in life. Such

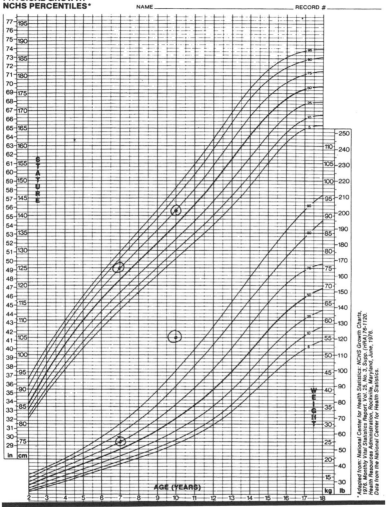

FIG. 2.1. Typical growth chart used to assess the height and weight of a child over a period of years. In this case, a boy aged 7 years weighed 25 kg (55 pounds), and was 125 cm (49.5 inches) tall, placing him at the 75th percentile for both weight and height. Three years later, at age 10, the same boy weighed 55 kg (120 pounds), and was 141 cm (55.5 inches tall). This placed him well above the 95th percentile for weight, but still at the 75th percentile for height. He should be evaluated for obesity.

information is being collected in the United States and elsewhere, but we will have to wait several more years for conclusive information to emerge.

Usually, when parents suspect that a child is obese, they take him or her to a physician. The physician may simply look at the child and, based on experience, agree that the child is obese. But not all obese children are so easy to diagnose. And some kids who may appear to be obese really aren't. They may be relatively taller than other kids their age, or their appearance may be due to an unusually large muscle mass rather than to excessive fat. So a better method is to weigh the child, measure the height, and plot these values on a common percentile growth chart. If both height and weight are close to the same percentile (for example, the 75th percentile or the 10th percentile) and there is no evidence of abnormal growth, we usually say that a child is within the normal range for both of these measurements, since weight percentile (the "ideal" weight) is usually fairly close to the height percentile in normal children. On the other hand, if a child's height is at the 25th percentile but weight is considerably above the 95th percentile, then this child's weight is more than would be expected for his or her height, and the child may be obese.

There's another way to diagnose and express obesity. Let's say a child's weight is 88 pounds, which is 33 pounds greater than his or her expected ideal weight of 55 pounds. By simply dividing the measured weight by the ideal weight, we can then say that a child's weight exceeds ideal weight for height by a certain percentage. In this example, dividing 88 pounds by 55 pounds gives a value of 160 percent. We can either say that this child's weight is 160 percent *of* expected weight for height, or that weight is 60 percent *greater than* expected weight for height. Children whose weight is 20 percent or more above ideal weight for height are defined by convention as being obese.

Yet another method which bases a diagnosis of obesity on a child's height is the *body mass index*, or *BMI*. There are several different body mass indexes, but the one most commonly used to assess obesity is easy to use and to calculate, is reproducible, and is a generally reliable index of weight for height. The following formula is used in its calculation: Weight (in kilograms) divided by the square of the height in meters.[2] For example, in the case of a child who is 122 centimeters tall and who weighs 48 kilograms, the BMI is 48 kilograms divided by (1.22 meters)^2, or 32. Body mass index can also be calculated with the following formula, which uses weight in pounds and height in inches: Weight (in pounds) divided by the square of the height (in inches) multiplied by 704.5. Like height and weight, BMI increases with age, and percentile charts are available for plotting. Most authorities accept BMIs greater than the 85th percentile as being indicative of obesity in children. Many growing children, however, may have weights that fluctuate both above and below this cut point, depending upon their age, and it would be a mistake to label such children as obese and initiate treatment. Children whose BMI exceeds the 95th percentile, as in the above example, are much more likely to be obese, assuming that body fat measurements are also increased.[3]

A disadvantage of the BMI is that it varies with frame size and also with leg length. Frame size is assessed by measurement of the distances between certain bony prominences, such as elbow breadth. Another disadvantage of the BMI is that is often hard to explain to parents and others.

In the remainder of this book, I use the term "overweight" to refer to the percentage of children, adolescents, or adults whose BMI equals or exceeds the 85th percentile for their reference standard age and sex and the term "obese" to refer to those whose BMI equals or exceeds the 95th percentile for their reference standard age and sex. The reference standard for adults is the sex-specific 85th percentile values of body mass index for men and women aged 20 through 29 years of age from the National Health and Nutrition Examination Survey II data (1976–80). The reference standard for children and adolescents is the sex-specific 85th or 95th percentile values from National Health Examination Surveys II (1963–65) and III (1966–70).

A final method commonly used in clinics to define obesity is to measure the thickness of the skin and fatty tissue with a special instrument called skinfold calipers. In children, this measurement is most often taken at a point halfway down the back of the upper arm, and is called the *triceps skinfold measurement*. Although similar measurements are taken at various sites in adults, reliable standards exist only for the triceps measurement in children. A child whose triceps skinfold measurement is at or above the 85th percentile is diagnosed as being obese, since values above this percentile closely correlate with total body fat. Measuring the thickness of the triceps skinfold is not a perfect technique, because the results are poorly reproducible. Quite often neither the same nor different clinicians obtain the same measurements on the same child. Despite this limitation, the measurement has been used in many studies to help distinguish obese from nonobese individuals, and it is most helpful when used in conjunction with the BMI.

Scientists can use several other methods to more accurately determine a person's body fat. We will discuss only one of these in detail, and simply mention some others.

The most accurate way to measure body fat would be to cut into a person and carefully separate and measure all the fat. The limitations of that method are apparent. We must rely on indirect methods instead. An indirect method of estimating body fat is to calculate the *percent body fat* by estimating body density. The density of a substance refers to how compact it is, and is usually expressed in the metric system as grams (weight) per milliliter (volume), or gm/ml. Body density can be calculated if body weight and the body volume are known. Weight is easy enough to measure. Body volume can be estimated by submerging an individual in water (Katch et al. 1967) and weighing the water displaced. Actually, the water doesn't have to be weighed, since we know that the weight of the displaced water, in grams, is equivalent to its volume, in milliliters.

Another way to estimate body volume is to weigh it out of water (in air), and then weigh it again while it is submerged (Siri

1956). Remember Archimedes' principle? Archimedes taught us
that the amount of weight a body loses in water is equal to the
weight of the water it displaces. This means that we can figure
out the volume of water a body displaces by simply weighing
the individual both in air and while he or she is underwater. We
then can calculate the body density by dividing the weight in
air by the difference in air and water weights, and we do this
in the metric system (kilograms per liter or grams/milliliter).
Knowing a person's body density enables us to calculate the
percent body fat.[4]

For interested readers, I have explained in further detail how
this test is performed.[5] Most very young children would not
cooperate for this test, although standards exist for children
as young as 7 years of age. Another drawback is that this
method estimates total body fat, including the fat in the nervous
system (brain, spinal cord, and nerves) and not just the fat that
determines whether we are obese or not.

Bioelectrical impedance (Guo et al. 1989) is frequently used
in clinical settings to estimate body fat. The equipment for
measurement is portable and inexpensive. The method works
because fat tissue contains very little water or dissolved salts
(electrolytes) and is therefore a poor conductor of electricity,
while other body tissues do contain water and electrolytes
and are good conductors of electricity. If certain assumptions
are made about the cross-sectional area and the length of the
conducting tissue, total body water can be estimated. In general,
the higher the percent body water, the higher the lean (fat-free)
body mass.

The principle of the technology is as follows. A harmless
low-voltage current is passed across the body. Resistance to
the current, read on the instrument, is determined by relative
amounts of fat mass and fat-free mass. Mathematical equations
are used to convert percent body water into an estimate of
body fat mass and body lean mass, which are incorporated into
easy-to-use charts. Bioelectrical impedance is not accurate in
severely obese people. Recent data indicate that this technology

is no better than triceps skinfold measurements in estimating percent body fat in children.

Other methods used to estimate body fat are found primarily in research laboratories and are expensive. They include total body water, total body potassium, total body electrical conductivity, and photon absorptiometry. Both computer-assisted tomography (the CAT scan) and magnetic resonance imaging (MRI) are used to estimate visceral fat.

In summary, the methods most commonly used to assess childhood obesity in clinical and large epidemiologic studies include height, weight, body mass index (BMI), and skinfold (usually triceps in children) measurements. More sophisticated and expensive methods are available and are used primarily in laboratory research situations.

How Obese Are Americans?

Let's try now to get an idea of how big the problem of obesity is in the United States. After all, if only 1 or 2 percent of the American public are obese, then the number of health problems due to obesity may be relatively small when compared to a chronic condition such as asthma, for example. On the other hand, if half of all Americans are obese and if obesity is associated with the health problems cited in chapter 1, I think most people would agree that we have cause for worry. We also need to know whether the problem remains virtually the same from year to year, or whether it is getting better or worse. We can relate changes in the number of obese Americans to matters such as total food and fat consumption, exercise habits, hours spent watching television, or cultural characteristics, and decide whether these factors might qualify as causes of obesity.

There are basically two kinds of studies used to estimate how many people within a certain population (for example, Americans, Canadians, or New Yorkers) have a disease or a condition such as obesity. The first is a longitudinal study. A relatively small number of individuals join a study at a particular time. At entry, people might be classified as lean, medium, or obese. Over time, those who were lean may become heavier, or they may remain in the same category. Persons who were obese at entry may remain obese, or they may become medium or even lean. And persons in the "medium" group may remain there, or they may become lean or obese. After a few years, investigators are able to get a good idea of how many people become obese and stay obese. These kinds of studies can be expensive because of the complex logistics of obtaining multiple measurements on the same people over a long period.

A second type of study more often used to estimate the prevalence of obesity in a population is the cross-sectional study. Here, a "snapshot" is taken of representative samples of a population. Naturally, this snapshot cannot be taken of all participants instantaneously. Time is required for those conducting the study to invite people to have measurements performed, to perform the measurements, and to inquire about eating and exercise habits. Consequently, a cross-sectional study may last for two or more years. The best-known cross-sectional studies having to do with obesity are those performed by the United States National Center for Health Statistics. The names and dates of the study, along with the age range of the population studied, are given in table 2.1.

The advantages of these cross-sectional studies are that the methods used in each are comparable, the participating individuals are selected from widely different communities, and the findings are largely representative of the entire population as well as of certain subgroups of the population, such as sex, age, and racial or ethnic groups. A disadvantage is that a different sample of the population is selected each time measurements are made. And these studies are also expensive, because they include not only weight and height data, but also laboratory data and information on diets, smoking habits, and other risk factors that affect the health of Americans.

Table 2.1 U.S. national surveys used for evaluation of trends in overweight and obesity.

Name of Survey	Abbreviation	Dates	Ages
National Health Examination Survey, Cycle I	NHES I	1960–62	18–79 years
National Health Examination Survey, Cycle II	NHES II	1963–65	6–11 years
National Health Examination Survey, Cycle III	NHES III	1966–70	12–17 years
First National Health and Nutrition Examination Survey	NHANES I	1971–74	1–74 years
Second National Health and Nutrition Examination Survey	NHANES II	1976–80	0.5–74 years
Third National Health and Nutrition Examination Survey	NHANES III	1988–94	2 months or more

With this background, let's examine some of the information about excess weight in American adults, children, and adolescents obtained from the studies listed in the table. Tables 2-2 and 2-3 summarize the proportions of overweight or obese children, adults, and adolescents in selected studies (Centers for Disease Control 1997; Kuczmarski et al. 1994; Troiano et al. 1995; Ogden et al. 1997). As you review these tables, remember that persons whose body mass indices equal or exceed the 85th percentile for age and sex *of a population reference standard* are referred to as "overweight," while those whose body mass indices equal or exceed the 95th percentile for age and sex *of that population reference standard* are classified as being "obese." The population reference standards are identified in the information accompanying tables 2.2 and 2.3.

Some of the findings of these studies are startling:

1. Nearly 35 percent of American adults 20 years of age or greater were overweight in the years 1988–94, up from 24.3 percent in 1960–61. This represented an overall increase of 44 percent since 1960–61!

2. Higher percentages of African American women than men

Table 2.2 Changes in percent of overweight* U.S. adults aged 20 years or more, by sex and race or ethnicity; from NHES I, 1960–61, and NHANES III, 1988–94.

Group	Percent overweight	
	1960–61	1988–94
Total	**24.3**	**34.9**
Men	22.8	33.3
Women	25.7	36.4
Non-Hispanic white**		
Men	23.0	33.7
Women	23.6	33.5
Non-Hispanic black**		
Men	22.1	33.3
Women	41.6	52.3
Mexican American**		
Men	—	36.4
Women	—	50.1

*"Overweight" is defined as a body mass index of 27.8 or greater for men and 27.3 or greater for women, which are the sex-specific 85th percentile values of BMI *for men and women aged 20 through 29 years of age from NHANES II data* (1976–80). The term "overweight" is used in this study since only body mass index was used and may have included some individuals having greater-than-usual muscle mass. Figures exclude pregnant women. Please refer to the text of chapter 2 for definitions of body mass index.

**Hispanics were not identified as a separate group in studies before NHANES III (1988–94), so comparisons with earlier years cannot be made for this ethnic group. Hispanics may have been included in every category in the 1963–65 period. Beginning in 1988–94, the categories "white" and "black" exclude Hispanics.

Table 2.3 Percent of overweight* U.S. children (aged 6–11 years) and adolescents (aged 12–17 years), by sex and race/ethnicity**; from NHES II and III, 1963–70, and NHANES III, 1988–94.

BMI Percentile	Children		Adolescents	
	85th	95th	85th	95th
All races				
1963–70	15.2	5.2	15.2	5.2
1988–94	27.2	13.6	26.6	11.5
Males, total				
1963–70	15.2	5.2	15.1	5.2
1988–94	28.4	14.6	27.3	12.3
White				
1963–70	16.0	5.6	15.8	5.4
1988–94	29.3	14.5	29.7	13.0
Black				
1963–70	10.3	2.0	10.4	3.7
1988–94	25.6	15.0	22.5	11.9
Mexican-American				
1988–94	37.2	18.5	32.2	14.5
Females, total				
1963–70	15.2	5.2	15.2	5.2
1988–94	25.7	12.4	26.1	10.8
White				
1963–70	15.7	5.1	15.0	5.0
1988–94	24.2	11.4	25.4	10.2
Black				
1963–70	12.1	5.3	16.5	6.6
1988–94	31.7	17.3	34.5	16.2
Mexican-American				
1988–94 only	33.2	16.2	31.3	13.8

*In this table, overweight is defined as body mass index at or above sex- and age-specific 85th or 95th percentile BMI cut points calculated at 6-month age levels. The reference standard for children and adolescents is the sex-specific 85th or 95th percentile values from the National Health Examination Survey II (1963–65) and the National Health Examination Survey III (1966–70).

**Hispanics were not identified as a separate group in studies before NHANES III (1988–94), so comparisons with earlier years cannot be made for this ethnic group. Hispanics may have been included in every category in the 1963–65 period. Beginning in 1988–94, the categories "white" and "black" exclude Hispanics.

were overweight in both time periods (41.6 vs. 22.1 and 52.3 vs. 33.3, respectively), and higher percentages of Mexican American women than men in 1988–94 (50.1 vs. 36.4). Yet the percentages of overweight white men and women were approximately the same, 33.7 and 33.5 percent, respectively.

3. The age and sex of a person are related to his or her being overweight. During 1988–91, 20.2 percent of men aged 20–29 years were overweight, but over twice this proportion, 42.1 percent, of men aged 50–59 years were overweight (data not shown).

4. The trend was even more dramatic among women during this same time period: 20.2 percent in the 20–29 year age group were overweight, compared to 52.0 percent in women aged 50–59 years.

5. Another disturbing finding is that, while the percent of overweight adults changed very little between 1960 and 1980, a 37 percent increase—from 25.4 percent up to 34.9 percent—occurred between the two time periods 1976–80 and 1988–94 (Kuczmarski et al. 1994). Significant increases took place in adults of all racial and ethnic groups.

6. More of our children are becoming overweight. The percentage (BMI at or exceeding the 85th percentile reference standard of 1963–70) among children (age 6–11 years) and adolescents (age 12–17 years) in 1988–94 was about 27 percent. *Nearly 14 percent of all children and more than 11 percent of adolescents were classified as "obese," an increase from 5.2 percent of children and 5.2 percent of adolescents in 1963–70.*

7. Overweight among African American girls and among Mexican American children and adolescents of both sexes tended to be greater than among whites, but these differences were not statistically significant.

8. The percent of black boys and white boys, children as well as adolescents, whose BMIs were at or higher than the age-and-sex specific reference standard percentile increased dramatically between the two time periods 1963–70 and 1988–94—by 12.1 to 15.3 points. Points for white female children increased by 8.5 and for white female adolescents by 10.4. But for African American

female children and adolescents, the group increased by 19.6 and 18.0 points, respectively, reflecting the racial differences seen in older adult women.

The same trends held true in the comparing of female children and adolescents whose body mass indices equalled or exceeded the 95th percentile, the cut point for definite obesity.

What do all these numbers mean? They mean that, since the early 1960s, the number of American children, adolescents, and adults who have become overweight or obese has increased dramatically. Of special concern is the evidence that African Americans and Mexican Americans are getting heavier at faster rates than white Americans. Why this is so is unknown, but what is suggested is that cultural factors may play a major role in the development of obesity. Other ethnic groups, such as some Pima, Navajo, and Cherokee Americans, also have high rates of excessive weight. The fact that our children are becoming heavier is a clear signal that preventive efforts should begin in early childhood.

Most of the increases in percentages of overweight children, adolescents, and adults occurred after 1976–80 (data not shown). Clearly, something has happened since that period to cause these changes, and the evidence suggests that the environment, not our genes, is to blame. We know that excessive weight is strongly associated with a person's age, sex, and race. What else could be happening? Are we, as a nation, consuming more food or simply more fat? Have we become increasingly sedentary, perhaps because we spend more time in front of the television set or computer screen than before, and because we spend less time in vigorous exercise? We know that obesity is strongly associated with certain demographic factors. For example, individuals in the Northeast and the Midwest are heavier than those on the West Coast, and city dwellers are generally heavier than those living in rural locations. Obesity is less common in people who have graduated from college than in those who have not finished high school. Members of low-income families, especially adult women, are more likely to be obese than their middle- or upper-income counterparts; persons of low income are also more likely to have limited educations and to be members of an ethnic group in which thinness is perceived as a sign of poor health. There are many possible reasons why overweight has increased, and it has been hard to separate out exactly which factor is the most important.

Many investigators have attempted to answer the questions of whether obese children are more likely than nonobese children to become obese adults and whether obese adults were also obese when they were children. Different measurements can be used: body mass index, triceps skinfold thickness, subscapular skinfold thickness, and weight for height (Garn et al. 1985; Serdula et al. 1993; Guo et al. 1994). These different methods of investigation make strict comparisons impossible. However, it turns out that use of different methods is a strength in trying to answer the questions above, since nearly all the studies come to similar conclusions:

1. In various studies, it has been found that about 26–63 percent of obese children (age 0.5–14 years) become obese adults, depending upon how investigators defined obesity, the age of the child at entry into the study, and the length of time that participants were followed. Put another way, obese children are at 2–6.5 times greater risk for becoming obese adults than nonobese children. The older the obese child is, the more likely he or she is to become an obese adult.

2. Recent information (Whitaker et al. 1997) indicates that if one or both parents are obese, the risk of a child under the age of 10 years becoming an obese adult more than doubles, regardless of whether the child is obese. Whether this effect is due to environmental or genetic factors or both is not known.

3. Not all obese adults were obese children. Both lean- and medium-weight people may become obese because of changes in their living habits: they get less exercise as they grow older, and they may eat more high-fat foods. Depending on the study and techniques used for measurement, it has been found that as many as 44 percent of obese adults were obese as children.

Summary

We have learned in this chapter that obesity can be defined in many ways, having to do with whether a person develops a disease because of excessive weight; whether he or she looks heavier than usual; whether certain body measurements, such as weight, height, the relationship between the two, and skinfold measurements are outside the "normal" range for age; and whether percent body fat determined by water displacement or other methods is excessive. We have learned also that obesity, however defined, is a worsening public health problem in the United States, since about 35 percent of adults and 27 percent of children recently were found to have body mass indices equalling or exceeding the 85th age- and sex-specific reference standard percentile. Finally, we have learned that obesity is a complex condition, possibly associated with a person's age, sex, race, or ethnic group, and that obese children have a high likelihood of becoming obese adults.

3. How Our Bodies Obtain Energy

A buena hambre no hay mal pan. (There is no such thing as bad bread when you have a good appetite.)

Gabriel García Márquez

Understanding how children and adults become obese begins with knowing how our bodies normally digest, absorb, use, and store food for future needs. The key concept is *energy*. Our bodies must have energy for carrying out fundamental life activities, such as thinking, breathing, eating, growing, moving around, and reproducing. In this chapter, we will analyze the steps necessary to obtain energy from the food we eat.

Acquiring Energy: The Essentials

Acquiring the energy to sustain life and to perform work and recreational exercise is a complex process. There are two central concepts that we need to become familiar with in order to understand this process. The first is that energy, the fuel needed by our bodies so that they can "run," comes from the food we eat. This food energy is converted to a form the body can use by the breaking down of dietary carbohydrates and fats, primarily, to water and carbon dioxide. Much of this energy is lost as heat. We will learn the basic concepts of energy utilization in this chapter.

The second central concept is that the whole process of the body's use of energy, including digestion, absorption, and storage of excess intake, is directed toward achieving *glucose homeostasis*. This means that *glucose*, the main sugar used as fuel by our cells, is kept at a relatively constant level in the blood at all times. The reason that glucose homeostasis is important is that glucose is usually the only substance used by our nervous system (the brain, spinal cord, and nerves) for energy. Other body cells may use protein and fat for fuel, but the nervous system uses only glucose, except in special circumstances such as prolonged starvation. If our nervous systems do not have glucose to use as fuel, then other parts of our bodies, such as the circulatory, respiratory, digestive, and excretory systems simply fail, since their proper functioning depends in large part on an intact nervous system. Knowing that blood glucose levels have to stay within a narrow range is very important to an understanding of how energy is normally obtained and used and of how obesity can occur.

Three terms will help us understand how our bodies take in and release energy. *Anabolism* refers to the process by which large molecules are synthesized from small molecules by the cells of the body. *Catabolism* means just the opposite: large molecules are converted, or broken down, to smaller molecules. And *metabolism* (which means "change" in Greek) includes both anabolism and catabolism: it is the entire process of converting energy from one form to another so that the body can use it. We will learn several examples of each of these.

The Digestive Process

All energy is derived from the sun. Plants and algae capture the sun's energy, which they store as carbohydrates, and animals ultimately get their energy from plants, which they store as carbohydrates, proteins, and fats. In humans, obtaining energy begins with the consuming and digesting of plants and animals and their products, better known as *food*.

We all know what consumption of food is, but what exactly is digestion? *Digestion* is the sum of all the processes by which the food that we eat is converted into a form that can be absorbed and used for energy. Since digestion is the first step in acquiring energy, let's review what our digestive systems—mouth and throat, esophagus, stomach, small and large intestines, liver, gallbladder, and pancreas—do and how they do it. Remember that our digestive systems actually communicate with our brains through a special part of the nervous system, the autonomic nervous system,[6] which signals the brain as to when we need food and when we have had enough. Our nervous systems therefore are of immense importance to the digestive process. In this chapter, we will concentrate on the digestion and absorption of *macronutrients*—the carbohydrates, proteins, and fats that make up the bulk of the food we eat—although *micronutrients*, such as vitamins and minerals, as well as water, are also critically important to life.

How Is Digestion Normally Controlled?

When we swallow, food is mixed and propelled further down the digestive tract when smooth muscle in the walls of the esophagus, stomach, and intestines contracts. Smooth muscle is supplied by nerves from the autonomic nervous system. These nerves are able to sense the nature of the food or liquid in the stomach and intestines (such as how concentrated the food is and how much acid it contains) and whether smooth muscle is being stretched because of the quantity of food. This information is sent to the brain in the form of nerve signals. Upon receiving these signals, the brain then instructs the autonomic nerves to stimulate smooth muscle to contract or relax and to stimulate the release of digestive enzymes (proteins secreted by cells which make chemical changes possible in other substances, but which are not affected themselves by the process) from glands contained in the walls of the digestive tract. All three of these—smooth muscles, autonomic nerves, and glands—work in concert to provide us with two very important signals: *hunger* and *satiety*.

We are all familiar with hunger. Without this deep-seated, automatic stimulus to look for and eat food, animal life as we know it would not exist. If we have not eaten for several hours, our stomachs begin to contract rhythmically, often producing what are commonly called "hunger pangs." Hunger is controlled to a great extent by the brain: stimulation of a specific area of the brain known as the lateral hypothalamus causes animals (including human beings) to eat. On the other hand, damage to this area can cause an animal to lose all desire for food, resulting in starvation.

Satiety, the opposite of hunger, is the feeling of satisfaction, or the absence of hunger, that we experience after a filling meal. As with hunger, the brain is important in producing satiety: stimulation of a second area of the hypothalamus, the ventromedial area, results in satiety. For example, even if an animal has had food withheld for several hours, if this area of the hypothalamus is stimulated while food is being offered, it will not eat. However, if the ventromedial area is damaged or destroyed, the person or animal cannot be satiated, but instead develops a voracious appetite, and, usually, obesity results. We will learn more about exciting new developments in the study of hunger and satiety in chapter 8.

What Does the Digestive Process Accomplish?

We won't list every step necessary in the digestion of food; let's just summarize how the process works. When we chew food, we cut, shred, and pulverize it, and our saliva moistens and lubricates it. After it is swallowed, food is further moistened by mucus in the stomach, and hydrochloric acid is added, which aids digestion of protein (and kills germs). The pancreas secretes bicarbonate into the small intestine, which neutralizes the acid, and enzymes secreted by the stomach, the pancreas, and the small intestine cause further breakdown of the food. Food that can't be absorbed, such as the cellulose found in much of the plant fiber that we eat, is eliminated in the feces.

Exactly what happens to the three major macronutrients—carbohydrates, proteins, and fats—during the digestive process? *Carbohydrates*, including starches and sugars, are found in foods such as bread, pasta, cereal, milk, and fruits. To be absorbed, they must be broken down into their simple component sugars—glucose, fructose, and galactose—by enzymes in saliva and by intestinal and pancreatic secretions.

Proteins, which are supplied in foods such as meats, fish, cheese, milk, and beans, are usually broken down by several enzymes secreted by the stomach, the pancreas, and the small intestine into their constituent amino acids for absorption.

Lipids, including meat fat, cooking oils, and the fats in nuts, cheese, and a host of other foods, are usually eaten in the form of triglycerides. They are acted upon in the intestine by bile salts from the liver and gallbladder, which help make them soluble in water, and by pancreatic enzymes, which further degrade them to their component parts, glycerol and fatty acids; these are easily absorbed.

Unless the macronutrients are completely digested, they cannot be properly absorbed by the body's cells and used to produce energy. To understand obesity, we have to understand the products of digestion and what happens to these products when they are absorbed.

The pancreas and certain specialized cells in the walls of the stomach and small intestine also secrete hormones into the bloodstream. *Hormones* are chemicals produced in one kind of tissue that regulate function in another kind of tissue; they travel via the bloodstream. Insulin is a hormone secreted by the pancreas. One of its functions is to help glucose get into cells. Gastrin is a hormone produced by the stomach that enters the bloodstream and regulates the secretion of acid and certain digestive enzymes. And cholecystokinin is yet another hormone released by cells in the small intestine that makes the gallbladder contract and squeeze its contents (bile) into the small intestine.

The Three Phases of Digestion

The first phase in digestion is the cephalic (the Greek *kephale* means "head"), and refers to the fact that digestion is largely under the control and influence of the brain. This is also called the conscious or sensual phase, because all of our five senses can play an active role in the digestive process. The second and third phases are the gastric and the intestinal, so named because most of the action occurs in the stomach and the intestine, respectively.

Cephalic (Sensual) Phase   We are all familiar with this phase of digestion. When we have not eaten for several hours, the smell of coffee brewing or fresh cinnamon rolls baking can focus our attention on eating. Our sense of sight also may compel us to seek food: television ads for pizza or hamburgers, recipes in magazines, and the presentation of a meal (how it is served, and how it looks on the table) are well-known examples. Children may think of food when they hear their parents describing a great pasta dish consumed at a restaurant the night before, or when they hear or smell popcorn popping. How food tastes and feels—whether it is seasoned according to our individual preferences, and whether it is soft or tough and chewy—may determine how much food we eat or whether we eat it at all. Finally, our past associations with the smells and tastes of certain foods and the environments in which they were eaten (such as the madeleines so brilliantly described by Marcel Proust in his novel *Remembrance of Things Past*) are very important: children may find a birthday party with hot dogs, potato salad, music, and games so enjoyable that hot dogs become their favorite food. A romantic evening meal with candlelight and wine may determine an individual's preference for a particular food for a lifetime. Real estate agents long ago came to appreciate the fact that the smell of bread baking in the kitchen can help sell a house!

On the other hand, we may lose our appetites when food is mentioned or served in certain emotional or unpleasant situations, or when meals are repetitious. We may be less hungry if we have just seen a film showing children who forage for food in garbage dumps, or if foul odors are being emitted from a poultry processing plant close to the restaurant we're eating in, or if we swallow a loose dental crown with our food. Having to eat military field rations for several weeks on end may not satisfy our hunger at all, and may permanently kill our taste for canned meats.

The central role played by our nervous systems in the digestive process, whether at a conscious level or an automatic one, is extremely important. Environmental impulses (sight, sound, smell, taste, and touch) that stimulate our five senses are transmitted by nerves to specific receptors in the brain, cells whose only function is to receive and process these nerve signals. The receptors then send impulses to the nerve cells in the digestive tract responsible for the nervous control of digestion, which activate, participate in, or terminate the digestive process. The cephalic phase of digestion is of particular importance in treating obesity, as we shall see later.

There is another important and automatic aspect of the cephalic phase of energy acquisition, and that is our "biological clocks," also known as circadian rhythms (from the Latin *circa*, meaning "about," and *dies*, meaning "day"). Circadian rhythms influence many body functions, such as our wake-sleep cycles, body temperatures, excretion of certain substances into the urine, and secretion of some hormones into the blood. For example, body temperature is generally about one degree Celsius higher when we are awake than when we are asleep, and the secretion of growth hormone by the pituitary gland is at its peak during a normal day when we are sleeping.

Circadian cycles operate internally in each individual, but depend on external (environmental) cues to set the actual hours of the rhythm. For example, our wake-sleep cycles are set largely by the natural light-dark cycle, the most important external time cue. Another important cue is meal timing. In the United States, most people are accustomed to eating three meals a day: breakfast, lunch, and dinner. Our daily schedules usually determine what time we consume these meals each day, and we learn to associate the eating experience with that particular time. If mealtime is earlier or later than usual, some of our body functions that depend on circadian rhythms can be temporarily disturbed and cause irritability or fatigue, as in the state known as "jet lag." For a little girl whose biologic clock has taught her that school lunch is always served at 11:48 A.M., a delay of 45 minutes can be catastrophic!

Gastric and Intestinal Phases   The digestive process ends a short time after food has finally been broken down into its absorbable components, and absorption then becomes the paramount activity. The switching of this process on and off belongs to the gastric and intestinal phases of digestion. They are discussed together because they are very similar.

What is (or is not) in the lumen (the cavity) of our stomachs and intestines largely controls the digestive process: both the amount of food in our digestive tracts and the composition of that food stimulate secretion of hydrochloric acid by the stomach, secretion of digestive enzymes by the small intestine and the pancreas, and excretion of bile by the liver and gallbladder. In this sense, the appearance or disappearance of food in the digestive system activates or deactivates the digestive process. You have probably already realized that the three phases of digestion—cephalic, gastric, and intestinal—can occur simultaneously during a meal and continue while food is being absorbed.

In summary, we now know how we sense hunger or satiety, how food is digested, and what controls the digestive process. To begin to answer the question "How does a person become obese?", we have to follow the digested food further along in the metabolic process.

The Absorption, Use, and Storage of Energy

The absorption of food and its use by or storage in the body are regulated by mechanisms different from those responsible for the breakdown of food to absorbable molecules. Over a long period of time, humans have adapted to frequent variations in two major factors in our environments: temperature and food availability. We can live within a wide range of temperatures, and we can live without food for a relatively long interval. Of course, adjusting to these environmental changes is not always easy or immediate or a conscious effort, but the biologic capability for survival is nevertheless present. This concept of how we are able to survive without food is critically important to an understanding of how and why obesity may develop.

For a moment, set aside the idea that obesity is a condition that can cause serious health complications, and think of excess body fat as a way to survive when food is scarce. When food is plentiful, we have more than enough energy for our bodies to function under resting conditions (breathing, circulating blood, digesting food), and also for conditions requiring greater utilization of energy, such as manual labor and recreational activities. Food energy which is not used immediately after absorption is not simply discarded by our bodies; it is stored in several forms, one of which is fat. Then, when food is scarce, stored energy is used as a source of energy, and we are able to buy time until food becomes available again. In this sense, obesity (storage of excess calories as fat in the body) is not at all an abnormal condition, but is an adaptive mechanism that has developed over thousands and thousands of years.

Let's learn how our bodies obtain and use energy under two conditions: first, directly and immediately from the food that we have recently eaten, and then from stored energy provided by food that was eaten earlier.

How Does the Body Use Food as an Energy Source?

What happens to glucose, amino acids, and fats after they enter the bloodstream? First, recall that dietary carbohydrates are broken down to glucose, fructose, and galactose. I will refer to all three from now on as glucose, since fructose and galactose end up being metabolized much like glucose.

Glucose enters the epithelial cells lining our small intestines, and is absorbed into the bloodstream and transported to the nervous system, liver, skeletal muscle, adipose (fat) tissue, and most other cells of the body. With the assistance of insulin, glucose enters cells and provides nearly all the energy required by the body for three or four hours after a meal is ingested. This is especially important to our nervous systems: without a constant and steady supply of glucose for nervous tissue, we become irritable and may have convulsions, become unconscious, and even die. If the glucose levels become excessively high, then glucose may be excreted by the kidneys into urine and lost as an energy source. Thus, blood glucose levels are tightly regulated by the body, as we shall soon learn.

Glucose can be transformed for storage in different ways by the liver and skeletal muscles. In the liver, glucose can be changed in one of two ways: it can be stored as *glycogen*, a large molecule composed of many glucose molecules linked together to be used later as an energy source, or a small amount of glucose can be converted to triglycerides. Most of the triglycerides formed in the liver from glucose are not stored there, but combine with specialized proteins called *apoproteins* to become water-soluble lipoproteins. These fat-protein complexes are then carried by the bloodstream to fat tissue anywhere in the body. On reaching the fat cell, they are acted upon by *lipoprotein lipase*, an enzyme made by fat cells and located in the walls of capillaries. This critically important enzyme once again reduces the triglycerides in lipoproteins to their component parts, glycerol and fatty acids. Most of the fatty acid molecules enter the fat cell to combine after activation with phosphorous-containing glucose molecules called glycerophosphate, forming triglycerides for storage. What remains of the lipoproteins moves on in the circulation to be processed by specialized receptors on the surface of liver cells. Glycerol molecules released from lipoproteins by lipoprotein lipase are converted by body tissues to glucose, which can be used as an energy source.

In skeletal muscle, which is any muscle attached to a bone, glucose can be used as a source of immediate energy, or it can be stored as glycogen. Whether in liver or in skeletal muscle, glycogen may be thought of as a small "bank" into which glucose is deposited and held until it is broken down by specific enzymes when it is needed for energy.

Proteins are broken down during the digestive process to their constituent amino acids, which enter the epithelial cells and are absorbed into the bloodstream. Amino acids are taken up by most cells of the body and used for new protein synthesis. Once the limits of protein synthesis have been reached in cells, additional amino acids are degraded by complex metabolic transformations to be used for energy, or they can be transformed to fatty acids for storage as triglycerides. Dietary proteins provide very little of total dietary energy under usual conditions.

Dietary fats (mostly triglycerides) are reduced in the intestinal tract to glycerol and free fatty acids, and are also absorbed by intestinal epithelial cells. Both glycerol and fatty acids can be used for energy by almost all cells but not by the brain. Glycerol and fatty acids can also be reconstituted in epithelial cells to triglycerides, which coalesce into large molecules that bind with apoproteins to form water-soluble lipoproteins known as *chylomicrons*. Chylomicrons enter lymph channels which transport them to the bloodstream, then proceed directly to fat cells for storage in the same manner that lipoproteins manufactured by the liver are stored, as discussed above.

In summary, dietary glucose not used as an immediate energy source is stored as liver or muscle glycogen, or it can be converted to lipoproteins for storage in adipose tissue. Amino acids are taken up by body cells and used to make new protein; the small amounts not used can be converted either to glucose or to free fatty acids when blood glucose and glycogen begin to be used up. Dietary fat is broken down to glycerol and fatty acids, molecules that can be absorbed and used for energy, or, if not, then once again reconstituted to triglycerides and transported as chylomicrons to fat cells for eventual storage as triglycerides. Fat tissue is thus a dynamic body tissue, since the constant exchange of fatty acids renews stored triglycerides approximately every two to three weeks.

How Does the Body Use Energy That Has Been Stored in Tissues?

We have now completed our discussion of what becomes of the carbohydrates, proteins, and fat in a meal that is normally digested and absorbed and of how these processes are regulated. We can use a common situation to summarize how energy stored as glycogen, protein, or fat is utilized.

Let's assume that you had dinner last night, slept the traditional eight hours, and had only a cup of black coffee for breakfast. When you arrived at work at eight o'clock, you discovered that your colleague who had been preparing a major report for your company's board of directors would not be at work because of illness, and you were being asked to complete the report and present it at four o'clock that day. You dropped everything to work diligently throughout the day, never stopping to eat. The report was ready by the deadline, you made the presentation for your company, and you answered questions until seven o'clock. You had eaten nothing for the entire day, but you nevertheless had sufficient energy to think about the form the report would take, select necessary information from the computer's database, prepare slides and handouts, make sure that the conference room was clean, and obtain necessary slide projectors. Where did the energy to do all this come from?

Within three to four hours after dinner the night before, your body had entered the postabsorptive zone, meaning that it had to obtain energy from nondietary sources, since no food was being provided. In other words, you had to cash in on one of the three energy banks—glycogen, fat, or protein—because your body had to maintain a normal glucose level at all times in order for your brain to function. This constant level of glucose was maintained by a process known as *gluconeogenesis* (*gluco*=glucose; *neo*=new; *genesis*=creation). "New" glucose was actually created in the liver from other substances in the body.

The first source of glucose occurred by the process of glycogenolysis (*lysis*=breaking apart). Remember the glycogen that was formed from glucose and stored in the liver and in skeletal muscle? It's not a lot, but liver glycogen became the first resource called upon to maintain normal blood levels of glucose during your fasting state. However, since there was only enough liver glycogen to supply glucose for about four hours, and since some of this was used for the energy of breathing while you slept, the glycogen stored in skeletal muscle also had to be used during your busy day.

In addition, the formation of fat virtually ceased during your fast, and existing adipose tissue triglycerides began to be catabolized to glycerol and fatty acids. The released glycerol, which constitutes about 12 percent of the weight of triglycerides, served as an important resource for new glucose formation. Fatty acids released by triglyceride catabolism were transported in the bloodstream bound to a plasma protein known as albumin, and were oxidized as a major long-term energy source. Fatty acids were also used in preference to glucose as a source of energy in some body tissues.

But the major source of new "building material" for *glucose* came from skeletal muscle, which was catabolized to form amino acids, the most important of which in your case was alanine (the amino acid mobilized in the greatest amounts when someone is fasting). Further catabolism of amino acids in muscle cells supplied most of the carbon needed for synthesizing new glucose during your fast. Had the fast continued for a few weeks, protein loss would have been very likely to have detrimental effects on your health.

The glucose obtained from the three above sources provided only about one-third to one-half the energy that you needed during your unexpected fast. So how did you get the energy you needed? Your body made a remarkable adjustment to keep your glucose level within a narrow range: the cells of the body actually decreased their dependence on glucose. That way, most of the glucose could be used by the nervous system, which, as you recall, uses only glucose for energy under normal circumstances. Your blood glucose levels were lower than normal during your fast, and the secretion of insulin was decreased, but the secretion of glucagon was increased, as will be explained in the next section. Furthermore, during fasting the formation of active thyroid hormone was reduced, which lowered the energy requirements of your body by as much as 25 percent.

How the Use of Stored Fat as an Energy Resource Is Regulated

Since we are interested in obesity, let's briefly examine the ways by which the body regulates the catabolism of adipose tissue fat. Because insulin is such an important player in fat metabolism, as well as in glucose metabolism, we will discuss it first.

Insulin is produced by highly specialized cells in the pancreas called beta cells, and is the most important regulator of energy production and utilization in the body. Insulin is normally released from the pancreas in response to increased blood glucose levels, which always happens after we eat. The pancreatic beta cells sense this increased level of glucose in the bloodstream and secrete insulin in response. Insulin is carried to most cells of the body (nervous tissue and the liver are the exceptions), and combines with specific receptors on the surfaces of nearly all cells. This insulin-receptor complex makes it possible for glucose to enter the cell. Without insulin, glucose cannot enter cells in a normal manner, and illness or even death can result.

When insulin is secreted and the glucose in the bloodstream is used by cells, blood glucose falls. This decrease is detected by the beta cells of the pancreas, and insulin secretion decreases or may cease altogether.

Insulin acts to *oppose* fat breakdown, since it helps glucose enter fat cells, where it can combine as glycerophosphate with fatty acids to form triglycerides. Insulin also increases the activity and stimulates the production of adipose tissue lipoprotein lipase, thereby accelerating fatty acid entry into the cells and subsequent formation of fats. Furthermore, it decreases the activity of *hormone-sensitive lipase*, an enzyme manufactured by fat cells which initiates the breakdown of fats in adipoctyes.

The net effect of insulin is a decrease of blood levels of fatty acids and glycerol due to the increasing and maintaining of fat storage. In practical terms, when we consume significantly large quantities of carbohydrates, insulin is secreted, and fat breakdown virtually ceases while it is in the circulation. Thus, a person who is overweight will have a difficult time losing weight if he or she eats large or frequent quantities of carbohydrates.

Fortunately, insulin is not the only player in fat metabolism. There are other hormones that, taken together, serve as a "check and balance" mechanism to oppose the action of insulin, allowing fat breakdown under certain circumstances. We have already mentioned hormone-sensitive lipase; its activity becomes greater with low insulin levels.

A second major promoter of fat breakdown is the group of hormones known as *catecholamines*. Epinephrine and norepinephrine are the principal catecholamines involved. Epinephrine is secreted by the adrenal glands, one of which is located above each kidney, and which are richly supplied with sympathetic nerve fibers. When the adrenal gland is stimulated, epinephrine is transported in the bloodstream to fat cells. Norepinephrine is released from the ends of nerve fibers which supply fat cells. Both these substances combine with specialized receptors in the walls of fat cells to stimulate the breakdown of fats, releasing fatty acids and glycerol. Catecholamines also inhibit the release of insulin by the pancreas, and stimulate the secretion of glucagon.

Glucagon is yet another hormone that opposes the actions of insulin. It is produced by the alpha cells of the pancreas when glucose levels become lower than usual, and it stimulates the breakdown of glycogen to glucose and triglycerides to fatty acids and glycerol, which can be used as energy after metabolic processing.

Several other hormones, such as thyroid hormone, growth hormone, and cortisol, are vitally involved in energy metabolism. Thyroid hormone has several important functions, one of which is to help the sympathetic nervous system and growth hormone (see below) do their jobs efficiently. It also helps set the rate at which our bodies produce heat while at rest—the resting metabolic rate. Severe thyroid deficiency may cause growth retardation, puffiness, and some weight gain, but is rarely a cause of obesity in children. An excess of this hormone can cause a decrease in body weight, since it increases the resting metabolic rate. However, this fact does not justify its use in treating obesity.

Growth hormone is critical to a child's growth and affects metabolism in three ways: it causes new proteins to be manufactured at increased rates by all cells of the body, it increases the release of fatty acids from fat cells for energy use, and it decreases the use of glucose as an energy source. So its net effect is to promote new protein formation by using fat, not glucose, as the energy source. Deficiency of this hormone can cause growth retardation, while an excess can cause too much growth of the skeleton, a condition known as acromegaly.

Cortisol, the other major hormone secreted by the adrenal gland, also has important metabolic effects. It causes glucose to be formed from amino acids, and it decreases the use of glucose by cells. Thus, it helps maintain glucose homeostasis at the expense of proteins. Excess cortisol acts as a powerful appetite stimulant, and can thus result in surplus body fat. (We will return to cortisol and the brain hormone responsible for its regulation in chapter 8.)

The use of energy stored by the body is highly regulated by several physiologic mechanisms. The reason that I have explained some of the details will become apparent as we learn more about energy balance and about why obesity prevention and treatment depend not only on limiting dietary fat and total calorie intake but also on using stored fat as a source of energy.

Summary

This chapter explains how energy is acquired by our bodies from the various foods that we eat and from excess energy that has been stored in our bodies. We have followed each of the three macronutrients (carbohydrates, proteins, and fats) through the process of digestion. We learned that after digestion, foods are absorbed and transported in the blood to all the cells of the body. Once inside the cells, glucose first is used immediately as the fuel to meet the body's energy needs. Glucose not needed immediately is stored as glycogen, amino acids are used to synthesize protein, and fatty acids are stored in adipose tissue as triglycerides. These stored forms of energy can be mobilized to maintain glucose homeostasis when energy from dietary intake decreases or is unavailable. A complex regulatory system, involving psychological, endocrine, and nervous system factors is involved in maintaining a normal body weight.

4. Obesity: A Disorder of Energy

$E=mc^2$

Albert Einstein

In chapter 3, we learned that the major sources of energy for humans are carbohydrates, proteins, and fats. We followed these foods through the digestive process, and learned how their digestion, use as energy, and storage are controlled. What we want to become more familiar with now is exactly how energy is used by cells in the performance of their various functions, and how energy imbalances can determine whether a person becomes obese or not. The secret to understanding obesity is to learn how the balance between acquiring energy and expending energy is disturbed. This chapter and the next will help you see how this balance operates.

How the Energy Contained in Foods Is Used by the Body

Suppose you are served a plate of food. Instead of eating it, you take it outside, build a big fire, and throw the food into the fire. What happens? After a little sputtering, the food catches fire by combining with oxygen in the air, and it burns. Oxygen is critically important to the burning process. Carbon dioxide and water are released into the atmosphere as the fire becomes hotter using the energy released from the food. So instead of a nice meal of meatloaf, baked potato, green beans, and salad, you have carbon dioxide, water, a lot of smoke, and a few ashes.

What happens to the food in the fire is similar to what happens after the nutrients you have eaten enter cells. Take glucose as an example. When a molecule of glucose is completely oxidized, the energy that is contained in the glucose molecule is released, and water and carbon dioxide are formed as final products. About 60 percent of the energy is released as heat, some of which is used to maintain body temperature in cool environments. The heat cannot be used to perform biological work.

The other 40 percent of the energy is conserved in a complex molecule inside cells known as adenosine triphosphate, or ATP. ATP is commonly referred to as energy "currency," and is found in all living cells. Energy released from glucose, protein, and fat oxidation is transferred to ATP, which then releases it for particular tasks, including the production of fats or glycogen for storage. A large amount of the energy released from ATP is in the form of heat, so that only about 25 percent of the total energy from food is actually used by cells to carry out their functions!

All cells require ATP to carry out their functions. One of the most important of these is manufacture of proteins, carried out under genetic control. A second ATP-dependent process is muscle contraction; we would be unable to breathe, pick up a book, or move about without ATP. Energy provided by ATP also enables many substances to enter and exit cells: we are able to maintain constant levels of glucose and salts and to absorb food molecules and excrete waste molecules with the energy provided by ATP. For endocrine glands to secrete hormones and for nerve impulses to travel from one location to another, energy provided from ATP is absolutely necessary.

Let's talk about the different amounts of energy released when carbohydrates, proteins, or fats are broken down. To do this, it's helpful to define a term that you hear, read about, or use almost every day, the calorie. A *calorie* (note the lowercase spelling) refers to the amount of energy required to raise the temperature of 1 gram of water by 1 degree Celsius. Since much more energy than this is commonly used in the body's metabolic processes, we use the term *kilocalorie*[7] (or *kilogram calorie*), which means the amount of energy required to raise the temperature of 1 kilogram (1 liter) of water by 1 degree Celsius. This term is usually abbreviated in scientific publications as *kcal*, and in common use is often spelled *Calorie* (note the upper case). The Calorie is the unit printed on food labels that tells us the number of kilocalories per serving and on the screens of our computerized treadmills and stair-climbers that tell us how much energy we have burned up. In this book, I use the term kcal instead of Calorie.

Now, back to our question: how much energy do carbohydrates, protein, and fat provide? Burning 1 gram of carbohydrate releases approximately 4 kcal of energy, and burning 1 gram of protein provides approximately 4 kcal of energy. But the breakdown of 1 gram of fat provides more than double either of these: approximately 9 kcal![8] (Since not all of each macronutrient is completely absorbed and used for energy—some may pass through the intestinal tract undigested or unabsorbed—we frequently use the round figures: 4 kcal for carbohydrates and proteins and 9 kcal for fat.) Thus, over twice as much energy is released when a gram of fat is burned as when a gram of carbohydrate or protein is burned.

Storing energy from excess calories as fat is much more efficient than storing it as glycogen for two reasons: fat is more energy dense, and it also attracts less water. For example, fat stored in the adipocyte is nearly water free, but tissue glycogen binds almost twice its weight in water. Without fat as an energy reserve, we would normally weigh 25–30 percent more than we usually do. Put another way, to store 9,000 kcals as fat would contribute 1,000 grams (half a pound) to a person's body weight. But storage of the 9,000 kcals as glycogen would contribute 2,250 grams (over a pound) to body weight. This is important to remember when we explore energy balance in the following sections. Fat constitutes about 80 percent of the energy normally stored in the body. And about half the energy used by liver, muscles, and kidney comes from fatty acids provided by the catabolism of fats. So under normal conditions, fat plays a very important role in energy storage in our bodies.

The Basics of Energy Balance

We have another major concept to learn if we want to understand how obesity occurs: energy balance. *Energy balance* means that our intake of energy can be fully accounted for by the expenditure of that energy. This relationship can be expressed as a simple equation: energy intake=energy expenditure. This relationship holds true whether we are talking about the human body or an automobile engine. The first law of thermodynamics says that energy can't be created or destroyed. The energy that is used by our bodies for work may be converted from one form to another, but it is always accounted for by the amount of work performed by the body plus the amount of heat produced. In a state of energy balance, the sum of these two components—work and heat—always equals the energy that is absorbed into our bodies from the food we eat.

We have talked about heat (kcals) produced by the breakdown of macronutrients. Let's now think a little about work, which requires energy to be expended.

We perform two kinds of work: internal and external. We are all familiar with external work: examples include lifting, moving, and pushing objects (including ourselves) from one place to another, as in rowing a boat, climbing a mountain, mowing a lawn, sweeping a floor, lifting a sack of groceries, or typing on a keyboard. Different amounts of energy are expended for different kinds of work, depending on the weight of the object to be moved and the distance that it has to be moved. External work involves contraction of skeletal muscles.

Internal work means any kind of work performed by the body that does not involve the movement of external objects; examples include digestion of food, contractions of heart muscle, secretions of substances by glands, and the synthesis or breakdown of glycogen, proteins, and fats. All energy used for work, whether internal or external, is eventually transformed into heat.

So if we want to measure how much energy is used by the body, we must first have a way to estimate accurately how much of it is transformed into heat. This is important to an understanding of obesity, because we need to know whether there are significant differences between obese and nonobese people in regard to how energy is expended. Did an obese person use less energy provided by the diet before he or she became obese? Is the obese person destined always to be that way because his or her capacity to burn energy is somehow abnormal? Of the several ways to estimate energy produced by human beings, three will be explained here.

How Energy Expended by the Body Is Measured

The first method for measuring energy expenditure is known as *direct calorimetry* (*calor*=heat; *metro*=measure). In this method, a human subject is placed in a specially constructed small room with no air leaks, one so well insulated that no heat escapes or enters. Air and temperature are controlled for comfort. Water flows through pipes into and out of the chamber. The heat generated and released by the individual's body increases the temperature of the water in the pipes. The amount of heat released can be calculated by measuring the difference between the temperature of the water entering the chamber and the temperature of the water leaving the chamber. This method, although it is very expensive, cumbersome, and seldom used except in research laboratories, is quite accurate.

More commonly, energy expenditure is estimated by *indirect calorimetry*. Remember the discussion of your plate of food being burned in the fire and releasing carbon dioxide and water? It is possible to measure exactly how much oxygen was required to burn all the food on the plate, as well as the amounts of carbon dioxide, water, and heat generated by the burning. The ratio of the carbon dioxide produced by the fire to the oxygen consumed by it is called the *food quotient*, or *FQ*. A food quotient has been calculated for almost every kind of food that we eat, including corn, beans, squash, and tuna.

After a meal is eaten, we can estimate the amount of energy expended by cells in our bodies by measuring the same two gases: the amount of oxygen *consumed* by the body in burning the food and the amount of carbon dioxide *produced* by the body over that time period. When a meal has been eaten, absorbed, and burned, we can obtain a *respiratory quotient (RQ)*, which involves calculating the ratio of the carbon dioxide released to the oxygen consumed in the burning process. It so happens that the RQ measured by indirect calorimetry correlates very closely to the heat lost when measured by direct calorimetry! And if energy expenditure is equal to energy intake (in other words, if the body is in energy balance), then the RQ is about equal to the FQ of the food mixture that was eaten.

The FQ and the RQ are different for different foods: for glucose and other carbohydrates, they are 1.00; for proteins, 0.81; and for fats, 0.71. As we have seen, burning a gram of carbohydrates yields about 4 kcal, a gram of protein about 4 kcal, and a gram of fat about 9 kcal of heat. Thus, if a person eats a high-fat, low-carbohydrate meal, the measured RQ would be close to 0.71, the FQ for fats. If a low-fat, high-carbohydrate meal is eaten, the RQ will be closer to 1.00.

Why is knowing about FQs and RQs important to our goal of understanding obesity? For these reasons: if the FQ of an ingested meal is known (balanced, high fat, or high carbohydrate), then measuring the RQ can determine whether a subject is in energy balance after that meal is eaten, whether some of the ingested food is being stored ("positive" energy balance), or whether some of the body's stores of fat, protein, or carbohydrate are being used for fuel ("negative" energy balance). By using these two ratios, scientists can vary the nutrient content of food to study how obese and nonobese individuals oxidize it and to draw conclusions from observed differences.

The third method of estimating energy production is called the *doubly-labeled water method.* Its use, since 1975, has forced us to modify many of our conclusions about energy intake and expenditure which were obtained by less accurate methods. Its advantage is that it allows total energy expenditure to be measured in subjects outside the laboratory setting, even at home; its disadvantage is the expense. We have so little information about childhood obesity because it has been almost impossible to study infants and children using the two calorimetric methods described above. This method makes such study possible.

I will briefly explain the most important principles of this method of estimating energy expenditure. Like indirect calorimetry, the doubly-labelled water method is based on carbon dioxide and water being the end products of nutrient combustion. The process works like this: two special forms of water called isotopes[9] are created in the laboratory by "labelling" the two hydrogen and one oxygen atoms from which water is formed. Let's call these "type A" and "type B" water. Both of these isotopic forms of water look and behave exactly like tap water. After they are drunk, the labelled hydrogen atoms are incorporated into body water. As body water is lost in urine, sweat, and exhaled vapor, the total amount of labelled hydrogen decreases. Labelled oxygen, on the other hand, is incorporated into both body water and body bicarbonate, a chemical substance in our bodies that maintains a constant acid-base balance. It, too, is gradually lost from the body. If we know the difference in the rates at which *each* of the isotopes, type A and type B, are eliminated from the body, and if we can estimate the respiratory quotient (RQ) from energy utilized, then we can calculate the rate at which carbon dioxide was produced in the body over a certain period of time. Knowing the carbon dioxide production rate enables us to calculate an individual's energy expenditure over this time period.

I realize that this methodology is complex and not easy to understand. The most important thing to remember is that since scientists now can measure total energy expenditure in babies and young children as well as in adults, it will be possible to begin to explain some of the mysteries of energy disorders, especially childhood obesity.

How Is Energy Intake Measured?

Measuring the kcals in the food that people absorb when they eat can be a difficult thing to do. In laboratory settings, scientists estimate this energy content by measuring exactly how much of each macronutrient is eaten and subtracting how much passed through the digestive system unabsorbed. This is most commonly done by having individuals drink specially prepared formulas or by weighing foods. Careful observation of the participants is required for several days, and appropriate corrections must be made for any uneaten food. Studies of this kind are expensive.

There is an easier, although less accurate, way to get this measurement. The study participant agrees to eat only from food that has been carefully weighed and supplied by an investigator, and collects and returns what is uneaten. The uneaten food is also weighed, and the difference between the food supplied and what is not eaten is a close approximation of what the individual ate. A correction factor may be necessary to estimate what was absorbed. This method is more acceptable to most people, since they can live at home. But since the direct observation provided by laboratory investigators is removed, conclusions drawn from this data must be made carefully.

Finally, there is the *dietary recall method*. People are asked to remember all the foods and the amounts that they ate in the last day (or 3 days, or week, or 2 weeks). This method results in a serious underestimation of how much food has been eaten, especially in cases of obese people, and is no longer acceptable for scientific studies. For example, a debate has taken place in recent years as to whether obese people eat more than the nonobese. Based on dietary recall, the conclusion has been that there is basically no difference in the amounts eaten by each group. When more sophisticated methods are used, however, there is little doubt that obese people take in greater amounts of food, especially fats, than do the nonobese (Prentice et al. 1986; Bandini et al. 1990). The dietary recall method has been quite useful to therapists, however, in helping people examine and understand their eating habits and patterns.

What Do We Mean by "Energy Balance"?

Let's restate the simple formula that we learned earlier about energy balance: energy intake=energy expenditure. We have already learned a lot about energy intake; now we will find out more about what energy expenditure really is.

There are 3 categories of energy expenditure. The first is the energy that our bodies *at rest* use for "internal work": lungs expanding, heart pumping blood, kidneys making urine, glands secreting, and so on. The energy that our bodies use when we are in a state of complete rest is called, appropriately enough, the *resting metabolic rate (RMR)*. A person's day-to-day RMR changes hardly at all, but big differences can exist among individuals: as much as ± 20 percent is common.

The RMR is the rate at which energy is utilized by the metabolic processes of the body. It accounts for 65–75 percent of the energy expended by a human being who is lying motionless. For instance, let's assume that an average adult eats enough food to supply 2,500 kcal of energy after absorption. In a state of energy balance, in which none of the absorbed food is stored as glycogen, fat, or protein and none of the existing stores are catabolized, about 1,625–1,875 kcal are utilized for internal work.

Several factors can affect the RMR. Men generally have higher RMRs than women, but women's RMRs increase during pregnancy, nursing, and menstrual periods. An individual's lean body mass, as well as his or her fat mass, directly influences RMR. Growing children have higher RMRs than older individuals because they are using energy to make the protein required for growth. People with infections, fever, excessive thyroid or adrenal hormones, or who are exposed to cold temperatures have elevated rates. As we shall see in the next chapter, there is emerging evidence that RMR may be associated with race.

The second component of energy expenditure is known as the *thermic effect of feeding* (TEF), or *dietary-induced thermogenesis*, and refers to the heat generated by the digestion, absorption, and storage of a meal. How much heat is generated by a food and how long the heat lasts depends on the kind of food eaten. Most of the TEF can be attributed to energy needed to make ATP, which we learned about earlier. The remainder is largely due to the metabolic effect of catecholamines released from sympathetic nerves before, during, and after food is eaten. The TEF accounts for about 10 percent of total daily energy expenditure.

The third component of energy expenditure is the *thermic effect of exercise* (TEE). This term refers to energy used by contraction of skeletal muscles, and is a measure of the external work done by the body, accounting for 15–20 percent of total daily energy expenditure in individuals engaging in average physical activity in Western societies. However, TEE represents the discretionary component of total energy expenditure, since individuals can consciously determine their levels of physical activity. Simply tensing the muscles while one is lying quietly can raise the metabolic rate slightly above the resting level. On the other hand, the intense muscle contraction required for vigorous exercise, such as competitive soccer, rowing, or basketball, can cause the overall metabolic rate to increase to more than 15 times the normal RMR. Table 4.1 lists the kcal of energy expended per hour by engaging in various forms of exercise. The impact of physical exercise on total daily energy expenditure (and therefore energy balance) can be difficult to assess outside laboratory settings, or unless the doubly-labeled water technique is used to estimate total energy expenditure. This is because people differ greatly in the frequency, duration, and vigor with which they participate in various physical activities, to say nothing of the accuracy with which they recall these factors.

We can now restate our energy balance equation in this way: energy intake = energy expenditure, or energy intake = resting metabolic rate (RMR) + thermic effect of feeding (TEF) + thermic effect of exercise (TEE). Since the TEF is a relatively minor component of total energy expenditure under usual circumstances, and since TEE is largely discretionary, the RMR has been the category studied most often in an effort to determine whether differences in energy expenditure exist between obese and nonobese individuals.

Because of all the variables affecting energy expenditure, such as age, sex, prior physical conditioning level, and cold exposure, the RMR is usually indexed to a person's lean (fat-free) body mass. Indexing means that one value is expressed in terms of a second value. For example, RMR can be expressed in absolute terms, such as the absolute total number of kcals used by a person per day. This may give us a number for an individual, but the RMR numbers of different people may not be easy to compare because of differences such as those mentioned above. However, when energy expenditure is expressed in terms of

Table 4.1 Hourly energy expenditure (in kcal) of a 70-kg man during different types of activity (adapted from Guyton 1981, 883).

Physical activity	kcal per hour
Sleeping	65
Standing in a relaxed manner	100
Walking slowly	200
Sawing wood	480
Swimming	500
Running (5.3 miles/hour)	570
Walking up stairs	1100

a person's lean body mass (i.e., kcal energy per kilogram of fat-free mass), these differences are practically eliminated, and meaningful comparisons can be made among individuals and groups.

We will discuss the measures of energy expenditure in more detail when we try to answer the question "Do obese people have abnormal energy expenditure?" in the following chapter.

Substrate Oxidation and Body Metabolism

One other factor closely related to energy balance can be important in keeping our weight at a constant level, and that is the relative amounts of fats and carbohydrates we consume (Flatt 1995). A person's weight is determined primarily by the intake and use of carbohydrates and fats as energy, since protein supplies only a small fraction of total dietary energy, being used preferentially for replacement of body proteins. Since most meals supply more carbohydrates than can be utilized for immediate energy needs, most of the glucose formed by the breakdown of carbohydrates is stored as glycogen in the liver and muscles. Very little dietary carbohydrate is converted by the liver to fat, assuming that meals contain carbohydrates, fats, and proteins. In fact, Acheson and coinvestigators have shown that, after a 500 gram (about 1 pound) meal of carbohydrates was fed to human adult subjects, only about 9 grams of fat accumulated in the body over the next 10 hours (Acheson et al. 1982). So the majority of dietary carbohydrates in excess of energy needs are stored as glycogen. And as more and more glycogen is formed, the body draws more and more on this excess for energy needs by increasing the rate of conversion of glycogen to glucose. (We know this because after a high-carbohydrate meal, a person's RQ remains at about 1.0 for a long time.)

One must consume very large amounts of carbohydrates for 2 to 3 days before the carbohydrates begin to be converted to fat by the liver (see chapter 3). On the other hand, since glucose intake stimulates the pancreas to secrete insulin, and since insulin inhibits the breakdown of adipose tissue triglycerides to glycerol and fatty acid, the amount and kind of carbohydrates consumed, simple or complex (see note 10), is an important determinant of how much fat *remains* on our bodies.

What happens when the amount of fat consumed exceeds the body's energy needs? Is excess dietary fat oxidized as an immediate energy source, thus decreasing the body's dependence on carbohydrates and proteins? Apparently not. *Fat intake has very little influence on fat oxidation* (Swinburn et al. 1993). Adding a 50-gram supplement of fat to an otherwise calorically balanced meal does not affect the amounts of carbohydrates or proteins oxidized as energy sources. The more fat we eat, the more we store in adipose tissue. Unlike carbohydrate and protein energy balance, fat balance is poorly regulated by the body. If a person's diet over several months and years contains relatively high amounts of fat, excess fat is far more likely to be stored as fat than it is to be burned as an immediate energy source, and obesity may be the result. Fat balance can be achieved only if we use the fat that we eat as an energy source.

In terms of energy intake and expenditure, body weight remains constant over a long period of time if the average RQ is equal to the average FQ; i.e., if we burn the carbohydrate and fat energy in the food that we eat. In the words of Dr. J. P. Flatt: "Do not eat more fat than you oxidize, considering your exercise habits. Exercise enough to burn as much fat as you eat" (Flatt 1993).

Summary

We now have most of the background information necessary to understand why people become obese. Here are the key concepts that we have learned in chapters 3 and 4:

1. All energy that drives our body functions comes from food that is eaten, digested, and absorbed.

2. After absorption, some food is used immediately for energy needs, and some of it is stored as glycogen or fat or is used to manufacture proteins. If weight is to remain stable for long periods of time, two conditions are necessary: the expenditure of energy must be about equal to the intake of energy, and the amount and composition of the fuel burned must be about the same as the amount and composition absorbed from a meal.

3. The three components of energy expended by our bodies are the resting metabolic rate (RMR), which is the energy expended in the fasting, sedentary state; the thermic effect of feeding (TEF), which is the energy used to digest and store food; and the thermic effect of exercise (TEE), which is the energy expended by external work.

4. The body maintains a relatively constant blood level of glucose, the major energy source for the central nervous system, by converting stored nutrients to glucose when necessary.

5. The energy released by the oxidation of each of the 3 macronutrients is as follows: carbohydrates and protein, 4 kcal per gram; fats (triglycerides), 9 kcal per gram. Fat is the most efficient energy storage molecule.

6. The amount of energy our bodies use can be measured directly as heat expended, or it can be calculated on the basis of oxygen consumed and carbon dioxide produced.

5. Some Factors That May Determine Obesity

Genetics is to biology what the atomic theory is to the physical sciences.

Dr. Victor A. McKusick, *Human Genetics*

In this chapter, we will use the energy equation to help organize our ideas about the possible ways in which obesity can develop. In some cases, we will discuss the clues that help answer the question "Is obesity inherited?" A leading theory addressing this question is that obesity probably results from an interaction of our genes with our environment. We become obese only if we have certain genes *and* if our energy intake is greater than our energy expenditure. We know a lot about how environment influences the development of obesity, and the goal of intensive research that is presently being done is to identify and characterize the genes that better explain the role of our nervous systems, hormones, enzymes, and other regulatory mechanisms in this process. We will learn more about this exciting area of inquiry in chapter 8.

For our discussion, remember that different researchers may have examined different phenotypes (from the Greek words *phainein* ["display"] and *typos* ["model"], meaning what a person looks like) in their obesity research. In addition, some may have measured total or regional body fat, others body mass index, others skinfold thickness, others resting metabolic rate, and still others a combination of these variables. At present, no specific genotype (meaning a clearly identified gene or group of genes) has been shown to be associated with any obesity phenotype.

We could make this chapter a short one by restating what you already know: obesity develops because energy intake is greater than energy expenditure, and the energy equation is not balanced. A net storage of food takes place. We express this in terms of our energy balance equation this way: energy intake = RMR + TEF + TEE + food stored, and by convention say that the individual is in "positive fat balance," since fat is very likely being stored. But if we left our discussion at this point, we would ignore information that helps us understand *why* intake is greater than expenditure, or *why* expenditure is less than intake, and *how* we might be able to prevent and treat obesity.

It will be useful to organize our discussion around a simple model of how obesity might occur. One of the most practical and helpful models is the one proposed by Dr. James Hill, Dr. Michael Pagliassotti, and Dr. John Peters (Hill et al. 1994). I will modify this model slightly but still refer to it as "the Hill model." According to this model, "[T]he genotype [of an individual] defines the boundary conditions or capacity of the system to respond to the environment. Nongenetic factors determine at what point within these boundaries the system operates. In other words, the genotype determines what can happen and the environment determines what does happen" (36).

The Hill model assumes that the two human characteristics of greatest interest, behavior and metabolism, have both genetic and nongenetic determinants. For example, an individual's *behavioral phenotype*, based on both genetic and nongenetic factors, may explain how much and what kind of foods are eaten, or how long and how hard he or she exercises. In addition, this model assumes that specific eating and physical activity behaviors of different people come from interactions between their individual behavioral phenotypes and, among other things, (a) their states of hunger or satiety, (b) the availability and appearance of food, and (c) the necessity for physical exercise (including physical labor). One person may prefer sedentary work activity, such as reading or working in an office, get little exercise, and nibble on snacks all day. Another may prefer the outdoor life, perhaps working as a tennis or golf pro or as a forest ranger, and may eat fruits, salads, fresh vegetables, rice, and very little meat. A person's eating and physical activity practices are likely to be closely connected to what he or she considers important or enjoys doing. There may be literally thousands of things that identify us as individuals, including food preferences, the speed at which we eat, and our exercise habits. In this sense, obesity cannot be called a "disease" in the sense that pneumonia or cystic fibrosis or diabetes are diseases. Obesity might well be the result of an individual's personal preferences and of how easy it is to practice these preferences in his or her environment. That's why the treatment of obesity may differ from person to person.

In the same way, a person's *metabolic phenotype* may depend on both genetic and nongenetic factors for its expression. For example, recent evidence suggests that African American women burn slightly fewer kcals when sitting still than white women do, so that more kcals are available for storage (Foster et al. 1997). If this is eventually shown to be true, it might at least partially explain why about 52 percent of African American women are obese, compared to 34 percent of white women.

Combining behavioral and metabolic phenotypes gives us the *functional phenotype* in the Hill model. The interaction of our functional phenotype with a particular set of nutritional and environmental conditions may determine what our body weight and composition will be. This idea has been referred to as the *set point theory*. Based largely on information collected from experiments with animals, the theory proposes that each individual has a unique metabolic set point, much as there are temperature, blood pressure, and blood glucose set points. The thinking goes that, for any individual, relatively constant body weight and composition are maintained if average energy expenditure is equivalent to average energy intake. This is because the body tries to "correct" short-term changes in weight. For example, if we overeat during a holiday season, we may gain a pound or two. To compensate for this, energy expenditure increases: resting metabolic rates increase (since we have put on additional muscle mass as well as fat mass); our desire for physical activity temporarily increases; our desire for food declines and we eat less (based on our behavioral phenotype); and body weight returns to its previous level. If these compensatory mechanisms are not brought into play, and we continue to eat at the same higher level, then we begin to store energy as fat, and a new set point eventually may be established. Similarly, if calorie intake is restricted, energy expenditure decreases, the search for food intensifies, intake of food increases, and body weight increases to its previous level. We will discuss these built-in "corrective measures" for weight fluctuations in more detail later in this chapter.

The set point theory has received attention in the past because of the well-known observation that many, if not most, obese individuals usually regain lost weight, while many nonobese people seem to be able to eat whatever they want yet maintain normal weights. It is a useful theory in that it helps researchers focus on the possibility that in some individuals energy intake and expenditure might be highly regulated, while in others poorly so. Recent evidence using the doubly-labeled water technique confirms that total energy expenditure rises with increases in body weight and falls with decreases in body weight.

It is not possible to identify a priori a set point for any one individual. If this could be done, we might be much better able to accurately predict during childhood which of us were destined to become obese! However, the concept of a set point has little usefulness regarding children, since constant change due to growth and development is taking place.

Let's now examine some of the behavioral and metabolic factors (table 5.1) that might explain how obesity develops and discuss some of the evidence indicating that some of these may be at least partially determined by our genes.

Table 5.1 Behavioral and metabolic factors implicated in the development of obesity.

Behavioral
    Eating behavior
        Eating behavior learned in childhood
        Social influences
        Family structure and personal beliefs
        Characteristics and availability of food
        Appetite and satiety
    Physical activity patterns

Metabolic
    Resting metabolic rate
    Thermic effect of food
    Total energy expenditure
    Substrate (nutrient) oxidation
    Adipose tissue

Eating Behaviors That May Help Explain Obesity

Many factors in the environment influence human eating behavior. We learned about some of these in chapter 3 when we discussed hunger and satiety, as well as the cephalic stage of digestion, including the influences of circadian rhythms. Eating is both a spontaneous and a learned behavior. From the moment a child is born, he or she learns that crying is likely to result in a full stomach. In fact, early infancy is referred to as the oral stage of development. As children grow, they learn to prefer some foods to others. This might happen because of the types of food that their parents offer them, which in turn might depend on the parents' food preferences. As a matter of fact, not only dietary habits but also total calorie and nutrient intake have been shown to "cluster" in some families. In one study (Oliveria et al. 1992) children having one parent who habitually ate foods with high total fat content were twice as likely to eat similar foods than were children whose parents had low total fat intakes. But when both parents consumed high fat foods, the probability of their children having high fat intakes was 3 to 6 times greater than in children whose parents had normal intakes. Without question, the dietary practices of parents can have a profound influence on the eating behavior of their children. But separating genetic from family influences is still a challenge.

What and how much people eat can be a major characteristic of a particular culture or group. For example, the French and the Germans usually eat their heavy meal in the middle of the day and a lighter one at night, while we Americans tend to have our biggest meal at suppertime. In developing countries, the percentage of obese people increases as income rises, and obesity may be regarded as a sign of economic and social prosperity. Almost everywhere, good food and plenty of it is the rule at weddings and funerals, where eating is a sign of our love, respect, and concern for others.

The structure of a family may affect the eating behavior of its members. In many American families, both parents work outside the home to maintain their income level and standard of living. As a result, their younger children must often be cared for after school either by another family member or in a day care facility, and a child's eating behavior may be influenced by these caretakers. Grandparents often shower attention on their grandchildren by providing calorie-dense foods. When parents are separated or divorced, children may live in two households; often, the efforts of one family to foster good eating habits in a child are undermined by the other family.

Many families eat outside the home regularly. A parent who holds two and sometimes three jobs may have little time to plan and prepare consistently high-quality, nourishing foods for the family, and turns to the most convenient sources possible— the fast-food outlets, which generally sell obesity-promoting, high-fat foods.

A person's self-image and beliefs may dramatically influence eating behavior. Adolescent and young adult women, for example, may become so preoccupied with their body images that they avoid food altogether (anorexia), or force regurgitation of it after eating (bulimia). On the other hand, overweight African American women may consider themselves attractive (Kumanyika et al. 1993).

The characteristics of certain foods may also influence a person's choices. Basic taste preferences, such as those for sweetness, sourness, and bitterness, vary greatly among people, and may be genetically determined (Drewnowski et al. 1995.) Much more research is necessary before taste preferences can be associated with food preferences.

Food is probably more available in the United States than in any other country. Convenience restaurants and fast-food chains are frequently open 24 hours a day, and many serve large quantities of inexpensive, but often high-fat, food. Government programs such as those providing food stamps and school lunches and breakfasts, as well as the Supplemental Food Program for Women, Infants, and Children (WIC), have made food readily available to most low-income children and their families.

Do Exercise Behaviors Explain Obesity?

Environmental influences have profound effects on people's exercise behavior. The nature of work performed by Americans has undergone dramatic changes in this century. An explosion of labor-saving technologies has led to a decrease in physical activity and to an increase in sedentary work habits. We have learned to depend on the automobile, the tractor, the mechanical crop picker, the washing machine, the airplane, and the computer to reduce to a matter of hours, minutes, or seconds the time required to complete a task which used to take days or weeks. But the trade-off is that we have fewer naturally occurring opportunities for vigorous physical activity and have to compensate for this situation by joining fitness clubs or by somehow finding time to walk or run before or after our usual workday if we are to maintain energy balance (as well as good muscle tone).

Like food preferences, many exercise habits are formed in childhood. Young children who see their parents engaging in physical labor or regular exercise programs are likely to follow their examples. A 1991 study (Moore et al.) found that when both parents of children were physically active, the children were 6 times more likely to be active than if both parents were inactive.

Some children, especially those in low-income families, have less opportunity for physical activity than what would be considered normal. Children who live in unsafe neighborhoods, for example, may not be able to play outside after they come home from school.

As children get older, they become much less likely to engage in regular and vigorous exercise for reasons including increased academic, work, and social commitments or school situations such as lack of physical education classes due to insufficient funds or substitution of nonphysical activities (for example, classroom or study hall sessions) for physical ones. Schools also may place greater emphasis on academic achievement than on physical activity or fitness, and may delegate responsibility for physical development to families. But some parents may not realize the importance of physical exercise to their children's well-being, as well as to their own. Other families may recognize the value of regular exercise, but feel helpless to create community or school programs that guarantee it.

Thus, while a child may be genetically or functionally inclined to engage in vigorous exercise, environmental conditions frequently determine whether such activity will take place.

Separating Genetic from Environmental Influences in Families

It should be apparent in the above discussion that families bear a major responsibility for a child's eating habits and physical activity practices. A child and other members of the family are likely to eat the same food at home and to have similar physical activity levels. Trying to find out how much eating and exercise behavior is genetically determined, how much is influenced by the environment, and whether either of these causes obesity in children is a complex task.

To study the relative contributions of genetic and family influences on the development of obesity, researchers have used indirect methods to make comparisons of obesity between children and their parents or siblings, between children and nonfamily members, between adopted children and their adoptive and biological parents, between identical and fraternal twins, and between twins who have grown up in different households (Börjeson 1976; Stunkard et al. 1986; Stunkard et al. 1986; Bouchard et al. 1990; Stunkard et al. 1990). Most of these kinds of studies have used body mass indices or skinfold thicknesses, neither of which is exact, as measures of body fat. Few have made comparisons in families by estimating body fat through the use of body density studies. But while we do not have the final answer about genetic and family influences on obesity, compelling evidence exists that both are important.

In the following sections, we will examine some of the possible ways in which people might become obese, taking into consideration some of the evidence that attributes an individual's obesity to genetic causes.

Could Obesity Be Caused by Abnormalities of Energy Expenditure?

Let's restate the above question this way: "Do some people become obese because they require *less* energy than nonobese people to drive basic body functions, so that *more* energy is available for storage as fat?" We can try to answer this question by first examining in detail an important study reported in 1995 that compared rates of energy expenditure between obese and nonobese adults. We will then look at additional evidence to try to determine whether children might have abnormalities of energy expenditure.

Dr. Rudolph Leibel and his associates (Leibel et al. 1995) were interested in how temporary increases or decreases in body weight affected the three components of energy expenditure: the resting metabolic rate (RMR), the thermic effect of feeding (TEF), and total energy expenditure. They were especially interested in whether differences in energy expenditure could be detected regarding obese and nonobese individuals. To answer this question, they selected two groups of people: the first consisted of adult subjects who were obese and the second of adults who had never been obese. Resting metabolic rate, thermic effect of feeding, and total energy expenditure (using the doubly-labeled water technique that we learned about earlier) were carefully measured in members of each group under the following circumstances: (1) after entry into the study, (2) after deliberate overfeeding to achieve a 10 percent body weight gain, (3) after returning to usual weight by calorie restriction, and (4) after losing 10 percent of usual weight by further calorie restriction. Metabolic studies were performed only after each subject's weight had stabilized for 14 days.

At baseline, before any weight changes had been induced by overeating, total energy expenditure and RMR (indexed to fat-free mass) were higher in obese subjects than in nonobese. Think about this for a minute: if obesity is explained by abnormal rates of resting or total energy expenditure, wouldn't you expect these to be *decreased*, with relatively more energy being stored than used? Instead, this study found that just the opposite was true: energy expenditure was *increased* in obese subjects when compared to nonobese. These findings were consistent with other studies (Weinsier et al. 1995), and are explained by the fact that obese people expend more energy in the work of breathing because of extra fat tissue in the chest and abdomen, and also because a greater work load is placed on their heart and blood vessels so that blood can be supplied to the excess fat tissue.

What happened after weight gain or weight loss in the two groups? With a 10 percent increase over usual weight, total energy expenditure, RMR, and TEF increased by 16 percent *in both groups*. The opposite was true with a 10 percent loss of usual weight: these measures decreased by 15 percent in both groups. Thus, changes in rates of energy expenditure apparently do not depend on a person's amount of body fat tissue.

These investigators did not directly measure the thermic effect of exercise (TEE), or nonresting energy expenditure. Instead, they calculated this as the difference between (1) total energy expenditure and (2) the sum of RMR and TEF. Interestingly, they found that after subjects had gained or lost 10 percent of their usual weight, most of the changes in total energy expenditure were due to large increases or decreases, respectively, in TEE.

What do the findings in this study imply? First, that if an adult gains weight by overeating, the body attempts to return to its usual weight by speeding up the rates of each of the three components of energy expenditure, burning up the excess energy and thereby preserving the status quo. Similarly, if weight is lost by undereating, the body attempts to return to its usual weight by decreasing energy expenditure rates. The above is true regardless of whether a person is obese or nonobese. Because of this remarkable process, body weight in adults is normally stable for long periods of time.

The second implication of this study relates to the clinical management of obesity. Obese adults who try to lose weight are, in effect, trying to defy the laws of nature! It is "natural" to regain lost weight, because our metabolic processes slow down in an attempt to conserve energy. We also become hungry and feel bad when we don't eat, and these sensations stimulate us to increase food intake and return to our usual energy expenditure rates. On the other hand, when we gain weight, our bodies attempt a return to usual weight by increasing energy expenditure rates. However, some people find it hard to listen to naturally occurring satiety signals, so they continue to overeat, and obesity may be the result.

Are Energy Expenditure Rates under Genetic Control?

Some evidence suggests that RMR may be partially under genetic control in humans. In 1986, Dr. Clifton Bogardus and his associates, using indirect calorimetry, reported their measurements of the RMR of 130 subjects from 54 families (Bogardus et al. 1986). They found that 83 percent of the differences among all subjects could be explained simply because of differences in age, sex, and the amount of fat-free body mass. Only 11 percent of the observed difference in RMRs could be explained by the fact that certain individuals were members of the same family. For example, the average RMR differed *among families* by about 500 kcal per day, but the average RMR differed *among members of the same family* only by about 60 kcal per day.

Others have found more striking evidence that RMR is partially under genetic control. Dr. Claude Bouchard and his associates carefully studied many pairs of twins among French Canadians (Bouchard et al. 1989). These investigators postulated that the RMR should be closer to the same value in identical twins than in fraternal twins, since the identical twins have identical genotype. They found this to be exactly the case: the similarity of RMR in identical twins was about twice that in fraternal twins. They calculated that about 40 percent of the difference in RMRs was based on genetics, far greater than the 11 percent reported in the first study cited above.

Finally, two studies (Morrison et al. 1996; Kaplan et al. 1996) which used different methods to assess body composition reported that prepubertal white American girls have RMRs about 200 kcal/kg fat-free mass higher than do African American girls of similar age and sexual maturation, suggesting that the white girls were more likely than the black girls to burn energy rather than to store it. Similar studies in adults (Foster et al. 1997) have suggested that race or ethnicity might eventually prove to be an important factor in explaining differences between groups of people such as white adults and black adults. Unfortunately, the two studies in children cited above did not assess other factors that might explain the observed differences, such as cigarette smoking, most recent meal size, or usual activity levels. Like so many other intriguing ideas, an answer to the question of whether a reduced metabolic rate is related to the development of obesity will depend upon rigorous prospective studies.

There is very little evidence suggesting that either TEF or TEE are under genetic control. This may be because TEF is responsible, under normal circumstances, for only about 10 percent of total daily energy expenditure. Rather dramatic changes in TEF are necessary for the inference to be made that it is an important factor in explaining obesity. TEE is difficult to assess unless subjects are studied under direct laboratory observation. Like dietary recall, physical activity recall is an unreliable way to assess TEE. Dr. Claude Bouchard and his colleagues at Laval University in Quebec have done extensive work in these areas, and have concluded that TEF may be approximately 40–60 percent genetically determined, while genetic influences explained about 30 percent of TEE (Bouchard et al. 1993, 1994).

Do Genetic Differences in Total Energy Expenditure Explain Why Children Become Obese?

Dr. Eric Ravussin and his colleagues tried to answer this question by measuring 24-hour energy expenditure at frequent intervals over a 2-year period in 95 Pima American adults, and related measured total energy expenditure (which included TEE, the thermic effect of exercise) to the participants' weight change at each interval (Ravussin et al. 1988). To no one's surprise, they discovered that low rates of total energy expenditure were directly related to weight gain: the risk of gaining a significant amount of weight was about 4 times greater in individuals with low levels of total energy expenditure than in those with high levels. What was really interesting was that the other family members of participants having low total energy expenditure levels also tended to have low levels, and family members of participants with high energy expenditure levels tended to have high levels. This suggests that an individual's energy expenditure can be at least partially explained by familial influences, but does not clearly separate genetic from environmental effects.

What if we could predict which infants were likely to become obese children and adolescents? We could pay extra attention to these babies, thereby perhaps preventing that outcome. Such predictions may one day be possible. Using the doubly-labeled water technique, Dr. Susan Roberts and her coinvestigators measured total energy expenditure in 18 infants (children who had not reached their first birthday), 6 of whom had lean mothers and 12 of whom had overweight mothers (Roberts et al. 1988). They measured total energy expenditure at 3 months of age, using the doubly-labelled water method. They reported that 6 of the 12 children born to overweight mothers, but none born to lean mothers, became overweight during the first year of life. ("Overweight" in this study meant that infants' weights exceeded the 90th percentile of weight for length, and did not mean "obese.") At 3 months of age, total energy expenditure was 20 percent lower in the infants who became overweight than in those who did not. Body mass indices and skinfold thicknesses were also greater in the overweight infants, indicating that they were fatter as well as heavier than nonoverweight infants. This investigation suggested that low total energy expenditure could be an important cause of the rapid weight gain in the overweight infants, and that at least part of the lower energy expenditure in the overweight children was genetically determined. A later study by British investigators (Davies et al. 1991) could not confirm the Roberts study. The relationship of total energy expenditure to the development of obesity in childhood must await further study.

Can Abnormalities of Fat Cells Explain Obesity?

Throughout our discussion thus far, we have scarcely mentioned the cell that is of utmost importance to the development of obesity: the adipose tissue cell, or adipocyte. To store excessive fat, the body first fills up all existing fat cells with fat. If the amount of fat is still excessive, then new fat cells must be formed. Does the adipocyte play an active role in the development of obesity? Or is it just a passive bystander, serving only to store fats when the amount of energy consumed exceeds what is expended, and making fat available when energy needs cannot be supplied by carbohydrates and protein? A few clues suggest that the adipocyte may be important in the development of obesity. Let's review some of what we learned in chapter 3 about the role of the fat cell under normal conditions.

First, fats entering the bloodstream are transported to adipocytes where the enzyme lipoprotein lipase breaks the fat molecules down to form glycerol and free fatty acids.

Second, the free fatty acids enter the adipose cell to combine after activation with phosphorous-containing glucose to be stored as triglycerides.

Third, the breakdown of adipose cell triglycerides for energy purposes (lipolysis) occurs in the reverse direction: hormone-sensitive lipase breaks them down to release glycerol and free fatty acids, which will be used as energy sources, into the bloodstream.

Fourth, insulin is a regulator of fat metabolism. It facilitates glucose entry into fat cells, some of which may be converted to glycerophosphate for triglyceride synthesis. Insulin also increases the activity of lipoprotein lipase and decreases the activity of hormone-sensitive lipase. The net effect is to decrease blood levels of free fatty acids and glucose by increasing and maintaining fat storage.

Finally, catecholamines are released from the adrenal medulla (epinephrine) and from sympathetic nerve fibers (norepinephrine) to adipose tissue regulating fat metabolism by opposing the action of insulin. They stimulate lipolysis and thus increase the release of free fatty acid and glycerol for use as energy.

Thus there are several possible ways in which adipocyte dysfunction might result in obesity:

1. An excess of lipoprotein lipase or a deficiency of hormone-sensitive lipase, both of which depend on insulin for their activity, would be expected to increase fat deposition. Neither has been demonstrated in humans. Nor has any defect in the ability of insulin to interact with these enzymes been described in obese individuals.

2. The phenomenon of insulin "resistance" in obese adults has been intensively studied in recent years. In spite of high insulin and glucose levels in this condition, cells appear to have decreased responsiveness to insulin, so that glucose is not transported into the cell in a normal manner. Adults having excessive visceral fat often exhibit insulin resistance, and are likely to develop high blood pressure, abnormal blood cholesterol levels, and non-insulin-dependent diabetes. However, since insulin resistance also occurs in nonobese individuals, its role in causing or maintaining obesity is not clear.

3. Extensive research has been performed recently to determine whether defective adipocyte catecholamine receptors exist which cause responsiveness of adipocytes to the lipolytic (fat breakdown) effects of catecholamines, thus resulting in excessive fat storage. One group of French investigators (Clément et al. 1995) reported a mutation in one of the catecholamine receptors (the ß-3 receptor) in persons with morbid obesity. But since the mutation was present to the same extent in a group of nonobese control subjects, the mutation could not be clearly associated with obesity. These scientists speculated that such a mutation might be responsible for the capacity of an individual to gain weight, given the necessary interaction with environmental and behavioral factors. Recently, other French investigators (Bougnères et al. 1997) have reported that the breakdown of adipose tissue fat in obese children in response to epinephrine is

less than in nonobese children, and speculate that this might be a cause rather than an effect of obesity.

Summary

We have examined some, but not all, of the "leading candidate" mechanisms that might explain obesity. A strong genetic component exists in several of these, including the resting metabolic rate, and there is evidence that race, in addition to age and sex, may prove to be a determinant of energy expenditure. Behavioral factors, especially those shared with one's family, appear to be of great importance for the development of obesity. The degree to which behavioral factors are genetically determined will continue to be the subject of investigation. Of the metabolic factors that lead to obesity, excessive calorie and fat intakes appear to be the greatest.

6. What Can Be Done to Prevent Childhood Obesity?

Everything our parents said was good is bad—sun, milk, red meat, college.

. Woody Allen, *Annie Hall*

What your mother always told you was right.

Dr. George Bray, Director of the Pennington
Biomedical Research Center, Louisiana State University

Most of us would agree that preventing a disease is better than having to treat it. But in considering prevention of obesity, we should first ask, "Is it realistic to think that obesity, whether occurring during childhood or later, during adulthood, can be prevented by action taken during the early years?" My own answer is a qualified "maybe." My reason for this somewhat pessimistic answer is based on what we learned in chapter 2—that the proportions of obese children and adults have increased dramatically in this country over the past 35 years. This is a compelling, though indirect, argument that preventive efforts can be successful: these increases were unlikely to have occurred because of widespread mutations in such large numbers of people. The increased rates of obesity could probably have been prevented during this time if excessive food, especially fatty food, had not been available and consumed, and if the majority of individuals had been more, rather than less, physically active.

We learned earlier that many experts believe that obesity most probably results from the interaction of an individual's genetic makeup with the environment in which the person lives. Let's take as an example of gene-environment interaction a person who possesses some genetic traits tending to produce obesity: a taste for fatty and sweet foods, an aversion to fruits and vegetables, a reduced signal to the brain that he or she is "full," a decreased capacity to burn fat as an energy source, a preference to sit rather than move about, and so on. Not only must an individual possess the genes necessary for obesity to develop, but the factors or conditions which interact with those genes, especially an excess of food (fat and calories), must also be present in the person's environment.

Let's now restate our original question in this way: "Can obesity be prevented in American children and adolescents in the coming years, assuming that food continues to be plentiful, palatable, available, and affordable, and that the opportunities for energy expenditure diminish?" To try to answer this question, I have selected several areas in which preventive efforts have been carried out or in which a need exists for intensified preventive efforts: macronutrient intake, physical activity levels, school-based programs, government initiatives, family-based strategies, and targeted prevention in groups of children at high risk for obesity.

Are American Children Consuming Greater Quantities of Energy and Fat Today than They Did 20 Years Ago?

There are several sources of information on what adults and children eat, much of it easily obtainable from the Internet: the National Health and Nutrition Examination Surveys (NHANES), which we learned about in chapter 2, covering the period 1970–94; the U. S. Department of Agriculture's Continuing

Survey of Food Intakes by Individuals (CSFII), carried out from 1985 to 1994; and other smaller studies, such as the National Heart, Lung, and Blood Institute's (NHLBI) Growth and Health Study, which concentrates on preadolescent girls, black and white, and their families. These surveys necessarily rely on the abilities of respondents to recall accurately what they ate in the recent past, which we know is not the best way to estimate daily energy intake.

Between 1970 and 1991, data from NHANES and CSFII (Kennedy et al. 1995) indicated that the estimated total energy intakes of children aged 1–19 years remained almost constant, or even declined slightly during the latter years. Only since 1991 have these two surveys suggested that the total energy intake in this age group has actually increased. How could obesity have increased between 1970 and 1991 when total energy intake remained unchanged, or even declined?

There are several possibilities, but one stands out: among American schoolchildren, total fat consumed during this time period probably exceeded the 30 percent of total kcals recommended for utilization as a fuel. In fact, during 1989–91, it was found that total fat and added (refined) sugars made up 35 percent and 15 percent, respectively, of total energy intake (Muñoz et al. 1997). And as we learned in chapter 5, when dietary fat is consumed in the presence of carbohydrates and glucose, it is very likely to be deposited in fat cells, under usual living conditions.

Why would children be eating diets containing more fat in recent years than in the 1960s? They eat more frequently nowadays than in the earlier years, and derive more of their total kcals from fat-containing snacks. More meals are eaten outside the home (not including schools), commonly in fast-food outlets, and more families carry food home that has been prepared in restaurants, especially fast-food restaurants. In 1989, for example, an estimated 200 people in the United States ordered one or more hamburgers in a restaurant every second (Massachusetts Medical Society Committee on Nutrition 1989). In 1994–95, 57 percent of Americans of all age groups—71 percent of teenage boys—consumed meals and snacks away from home on any given day, up from 43 percent in 1977. Especially alarming is the fact that 40–55 percent of kcals in most fast-food meals are derived from fat (Borrud 1997). As a result of these changes in eating patterns, inadequate amounts of fresh fruits, vegetables, and complex carbohydrates,[10] but excessive amounts of fats, are consumed.

Is this trend likely to continue, given the fact that about 75 percent of American women work outside the home? Yes, because with many working parents, preparation of any meal, much less a healthy one, can constitute a major time commitment. Americans want to earn money for decent housing and good educations for their children, and will do what is necessary to achieve those goals. A trade-off is that our families' nutritional well-being may suffer.

Is the availability of highly palatable fatty foods demanded by Americans likely to decrease, given the fact that ours is primarily a competitive, market-driven economy, and that investor return is its predominant current driving force? Not very. Will food manufacturers and retailers step forward and voluntarily withdraw high-fat food items that are big income producers just because health professionals keep pointing to their association with increasing rates of obesity and its complications? Probably not. Yet many food producers and retailers have demonstrated sensitivity to public demand for low-fat foods in recent years by making such products available along with the foods higher in fat. Will the federal school lunch/breakfast program *really* insist on an average fat content of 30 percent or less in our children's school meals since being required to do so by the U. S. Department of Agriculture in July 1998?

The hope for obesity prevention is that as more Americans get the message that eating excessive amounts of foods, especially fatty foods, can result in obesity for many of us, people's buying habits will reflect less responsiveness to advertising of foods with unacceptably high fat and calorie content. After all, the market economy can work to the advantage of the public's health as well as to its disadvantage.

Are Children and Adolescents Less Active Today?

A logical question in the pursuit of an explanation of the recently increased rates of childhood obesity is "Have our young people spent less time engaged in physical activity and has such activity been less intense in recent years?" If so, then implementing measures to increase activity levels might help prevent obesity. Although data on physical activity levels and physical fitness over time are not as extensive as those on energy intake, several studies (Centers for Disease Control 1990, 1991, 1996; Pate et al. 1990) have identified some consistent patterns:

1. In recent years, schoolchildren's participation in all types of physical activity has decreased as they grow older. Studies show that 70 percent of 12-year-old children report that they regularly engage in vigorous physical activity. But by the time they become 21 years old, only 42 percent of men and 30 percent of women say that they are vigorously active.

2. About one-fourth of young people 12–21 years of age say they never engage in any vigorous physical activity.

3. Female adolescents are much less physically active than male adolescents.

4. Daily enrollment in physical education classes among high school students declined from 42 percent in 1991 to 25 percent in 1995. But enrollment doesn't tell the whole story: only 19 percent of all high school students report that they are physically active for 20 minutes or more in physical education classes every day of the school week.

5. In the 1990 Youth Risk Behavior Survey (Heath et al. 1994), more than 35 percent of students in grades 9–12 reported watching television for 3 hours or more each school day.

How can physical activity levels be increased in our older

youngsters? Is school where the effort should be made? Consider the following information before you answer this question:

1. While there is some evidence that pilot studies in schools can make a small difference in children's activity levels, there have been few reports of widespread adoption of health education curricula by school districts to extend the benefits of physical activity to all who are enrolled.

2. Schools often send mixed messages. On the one hand, healthy living habits may be taught in the classroom, while at the same time students are served fat-laden meals or placed in physical education programs which may stress competitive sports rather than participation based on the student's developmental stage. In some U. S. schools emphasis is placed on winning at games rather than on the physical development of all students. Consequently, those who are the best at physical activities are selected for sports competition, with the more average student being less likely to participate in a regular, vigorous exercise program.

3. Many schools have discontinued physical education programs because of adverse financial pressures.

4. If schools can't or won't bear responsibility for healthy physical activity for our children, who will? Barriers to physical activity and fitness are found not only in our schools but also in our homes and elsewhere in the community. For example, parents are often not physically fit themselves, and may place little priority on their children's fitness and activity levels (Moore et al. 1991). The 1987 National Youth and Fitness Study II Report (Ross et al. 1987) found that fewer than 30 percent of mothers and fathers of children in grades 1–4 said that they participated in moderate-to-vigorous exercise themselves 3 days a week.

5. At least one recent study (Gortmaker 1996) has implicated the sedentary behavior associated with excessive television viewing as a cause of obesity. The average child and the average adolescent watch television for 21–23 hours a week. Young people usually don't exercise while watching TV but do usually eat

something, and they get ideas for more eating from ads for high-fat, high-calorie foods.

6. Often parents do want their children to be physically active, but their neighborhoods may have become unsafe because of violence; they may live in areas without sidewalks or with heavy traffic that limits most physical activity; supervised after-school programs which include vigorous exercise are either unavailable, inaccessible, or unaffordable; or their work schedules do not permit them to consistently oversee their children's activities.

If obesity is to be prevented, all elements of a community must clearly identify the reasons why so many children do not or cannot have acceptable physical activity and fitness levels, and devise ways to correct this problem together. A starting point would be for adults to set good examples of physical exercise based on recent recommendations (Pate et al. 1995; National Institutes of Health Consensus Statement on Physical Activity and Cardiovascular Health 1995).

Don't Schools Teach Students about Nutrition and Other Health Subjects?

Let's expand our discussion about schools beyond physical education programs. Schools have been identified as the best places for interventions that promote healthy nutrition and exercise habits in children and adolescents. Over 95 percent of Americans aged 5–17 attend school regularly. Schools are children's "work places," where intensive contact takes place with adult teachers and with peers, where one to two daily meals are eaten in a socially acceptable atmosphere, and where basic knowledge and skills which promote productive interaction in society can be acquired. Physical education programs of some kind are frequently available, although they may have to compete with band, choir, study hall, and work-study programs for students' attention. So it appears that school would be the best place to undertake the prevention of obesity.

But schools may have one or more of the following constraints relating to health education and obesity prevention:

1. Lack of qualified personnel to conduct a curriculum pertaining to health education.

2. No requirement in the school district for a health education curriculum, much less specific obesity-prevention programs.

3. Competition between a program of basic health education and one concerned with more pressing social problems, such as adolescent pregnancy, sexually transmitted diseases, and drug and alcohol abuse.

4. The understandable position taken by many teachers and administrators that schools should be primarily concerned with educating children in basic languages, mathematics, and sciences, rather than providing a program of health education, an addition which might result in further overcrowding of the curriculum.

Many schools have probably provided nutrition education to students in courses such as those linked to physical education classes. But other approaches may be more likely to result in changes in health behaviors. For example, a document entitled *Guidelines for School Health Programs to Promote Lifelong Healthy Eating* (Centers for Disease Control 1996) provides schools with a plan for moving *away from* approaches to health education based on the teacher imparting knowledge to students and *toward* methods that require hands-on involvement and problem-solving by students. This widely endorsed publication contains several recommendations and ideas for schools to follow in establishing school-based nutrition education, including integration of school food services with the nutrition education curricula, the training of school staff who will teach nutrition education, the involvement of families and communities in school nutrition education curricula, and ways to monitor the progress of school health and nutrition programs. The emphasis is on involving children and their families in a well-organized, culturally sensitive nutrition education plan. I think that this document holds great promise for implementing health curricula in many schools.

Some schools have welcomed special demonstration interventions promoting healthy eating and appropriate exercise among students. One of these, the CATCH program (Child and Adolescent Trial for Cardiovascular Health) involved over 5,000 elementary school children in 96 schools in California, Louisiana, and Minnesota between 1991 and 1994 (Luepker et al. 1996). Schools were randomly designated as intervention (56) or control (40) schools. Interventions consisted of the implementation of specific school-based curricula for food services (such as limiting fat intake to 30 percent of kcals), physical education classes (such as increasing the amount of moderate to vigorous daily exercise), and the classroom (such as promotion of skills related to the making of healthy food choices), as well as home-based curricula, which provided health information to families and required evidence of parental participation and knowledge. Rather remarkable results were reported: fat content of school lunches fell from nearly 39 percent to less than 32 percent in intervention schools, compared to a drop from nearly 39 percent to 36.2 percent in control schools, and physical activity levels significantly increased in intervention schools. Weight changes were not evaluated. Without question, this landmark study demonstrated that very positive changes could be made in modifying energy intake and expenditure in schoolchildren under well-financed, well-planned conditions.

Unfortunately, thousands of other schools in this country may not be able to adopt the intervention curricula of this or similar studies because of constraints such as those enumerated earlier. The U. S. Department of Agriculture's requirement that, starting in July 1998, the total fat content of school lunches could not exceed a weekly average of 30 percent was another attempt to encourage healthy eating behavior in schools.

Can Government Help Prevent Obesity in Children and Adolescents?

An entire chapter of this book could be devoted to a discussion of the remarkable contributions of our federal and state governments to the health of this nation. I will mention only a few:

1. National surveillance studies, such as the NHES, NHANES, CSFII, and the NHLBI growth and health studies, keep the American public informed about the prevalence of obesity and its consequences, such as diabetes. Americans can be stimulated to action by information that affects their health.

2. The *Dietary Guidelines for Americans* (U. S. Department of Agriculture Web site 1995) and the Food Pyramid (fig. 6.1) specify the number of daily servings of foods, especially vegetables, fruits, and grain products, which can help a person maintain a healthy weight. These guidelines are used by dietitians and other

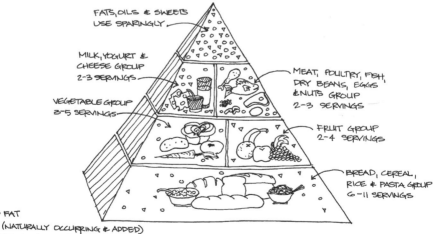

FIG. 6.1. U. S. Department of Agriculture Food Pyramid showing how often one should eat various foods to maintain health.

health professionals for nutrition education, and are based on sound scientific principles. They serve as a standard by which other government programs such as the school lunch/breakfast program are evaluated. The *Guidelines* was also used as the standard for the nutrition facts label, which gives the calorie, fat, cholesterol, and sodium content of most commercially sold foods in the United States. The providing of this information has greatly enhanced the consumer's ability to choose foods with desirable caloric and fat levels.

3. The U. S. government has also developed and widely disseminated the publication *Healthy People 2000: National Health Promotion and Disease Prevention Objectives* (U. S. Department of Health and Human Services 1991). The goal of this document is to improve the health of Americans by proposing specific objectives to be reached by the year 2000. One of the nutrition objectives, for example, is to "reduce overweight to a prevalence of no more than 20 percent among people aged 20 and older and no more than 15 percent among adolescents aged 12 through 19." Although that particular goal will not be met, this seminal publication acts as a yardstick with which to measure progress in many health-related fields, including nutrition. It is particularly valuable to state and local governments as a guidebook for the most important health issues among Americans, because it can assist in health-related policy and planning.

There has been and will continue to be involvement by government at all levels which may directly or indirectly help prevent obesity. Governments can provide funds for obesity-related research and education, can present facts about obesity to the public through publications and other media initiatives, can better recognize the proper development of American youth by placing increased emphasis on school physical education programs, and can help create incentives for the private sector, such as the food industry, to use the *Dietary Guidelines* and thus contribute to the better health of Americans.

What Can Parents Do to Prevent Young Children from Becoming Obese?

Dr. William Dietz, former director of the Clinical Nutrition Program at Tufts University, has proposed three critical periods in a child's normal development when obesity may be a threat: (1) the late prenatal period, which encompasses the 3 months or so just before birth, in which the number of adipocytes, or fat cells, markedly increases, (2) the period of adiposity rebound, which occurs between the ages of 4 and 7 years in most children, and after which both the size and the number of fat cells increase[n] and (3) adolescence, in which fat redistribution, such as increased visceral fat, occurs (Dietz 1994).

Overnutrition during the prenatal period may lead to an abnormally high number of fat cells, and an obese newborn may be the result. This situation can occur when the unborn baby is exposed to high levels of glucose, which may be the case if the baby's mother has poorly controlled diabetes. Obese infants born to diabetic mothers are frequently obese later in life. African American and Mexican American women of reproductive age are much more likely than white women to develop diabetes while they are pregnant ("gestational" diabetes, which usually disappears after delivery), and their children are at higher risk of overnutrition than those of white mothers. While any woman of reproductive age can, by entering prenatal care as early as possible in her pregnancy, help prevent obesity in her baby, special efforts should be made regarding minority women.

Prevention of obesity during the period of adiposity rebound, at adolescence, and at other times requires even more parental involvement. In my experience, the family can be the strongest factor in preventing obesity during childhood. The parent has the capacity to exert far more influence on dietary and physical activity behavior than schools or governments.

Most parents bring children into the world expecting to nurture, teach, and provide for them. Children are sources of joy and love, and parents normally are intimately involved in their lives. However, few parents have received instructions on what their duties are. Since the skills necessary to be a good parent are acquired by on-the-job training, most of us learn as we go along, and we do not expect to be perfect. Much of what we do as parents is influenced by interaction with our children: energetic and demanding youngsters are apt to elicit certain kinds of responses and quiet, easy-to-please children other kinds.

I doubt if very many parents sit down together after a child is born and say, "How can we prevent obesity?" We are more likely to be concerned that our children have normal appetites, don't play with their food, and don't have nutritional deficiencies. And yet, if 1 of 4 children in our country is obese, and if obesity can result in social rejection and psychological problems during one's childhood and in lower earning potential, reduced prospects of marriage, and health complications later in life, wouldn't it make sense for children to learn how to maintain a healthy weight as part of a practice of beneficial living habits? The establishing of such habits should be a vital part of the process of development of self-acceptance, self-confidence, and self-esteem, which happens at this critical time in a person's life.

There has been debate among investigators (Hammer 1992) in the recent past as to whether early feeding practices, including breast versus bottle feeding, the age at which solid foods such as cereals are offered, and overweight in early infancy (the first 6 months of life) unrelated to diabetes, can lead to obesity. After thoroughly reviewing these studies, the fairest comment I can make is that there is insufficient evidence to conclude that any of these 3 factors affects the eventual weight of a child.

Does this mean that parents have no influence during the period of infancy and early childhood on a child's future weight? To the contrary—this is when parents should begin to adopt and practice nurturing habits that can be continued into later childhood. For example, there is substantial evidence that parents should provide healthy food choices and allow a child to determine how much food is consumed, but should not necessarily project their own eating styles onto their children.

Naturally, parents want to offer sufficient food at mealtime and provide sufficient time in which to eat it. But as we learned in chapter 5, naturally occurring metabolic processes provide the built-in ability for children to decrease food intake as the energy density (especially fats) increases and to increase intake if calorie content of the diet is low. There is ample evidence in the health literature that the use of coercive strategies such as prompting, bribing, threatening, or using rewards in an attempt to get children to eat is counterproductive (Johnson et al. 1994).

In short, I think that the best advice for parents is for them to provide healthy food in accordance with the *Dietary Guidelines for Americans*, to allow children to eat from this selection only what they want, and not to succumb to the idea that a child will starve if he or she does not eat everything served at every meal. Children of parents who engage in controlling behavior at mealtimes may become insensitive to the natural signals that regulate food intake and determine weight. Here's what I advise parents to tell children who have reached their second birthday (not in these exact words!): "It's okay if you don't eat everything on your plate. In the interest of your good health, I will continue to provide 5 servings a day of fruits and vegetables, along with cereals and bread, and will try to limit your total fat intake to 30 percent or less of total kcals by limiting dairy products, meat, other fats, and snacks between meals. And, by the way, the rules are the same for everyone else in the family, including your parents."

Our goal as parents should be to help children assume responsibility for their own healthy nutrition choices and physical activity by teaching them to link nutrition to their physical functioning and well-being, to promote their knowledge of the nutrients in the foods they eat and the health benefits of these nutrients, and to allow natural, biological signals related to eating and physical activity to be expressed. And parents of young children need to provide examples of what is important by engaging in physical activity with them every day. In this context, it is not the prevention specifically of obesity or of eating disorders such as anorexia or bulimia that is the object. The goal is to create healthy eating and exercise behaviors as part of the child's overall development as a human being.

Should Children Who Are at High Risk for Developing Obesity Receive Extra Attention?

In chapter 2, we became acquainted with tables showing that during 1988–94, about 24 percent of children and adolescents exceeded the 85th reference percentile (1963–70) for weight, and about 12 percent exceeded the 95th reference percentile. Let's look more closely at specific groups of children in whom the prevalence of obesity is even higher.

In 1988–94, more African American and Mexican American female children and adolescents were obese than were whites (equalled or exceeded the 95th age-, sex-, and race-specific body mass index reference percentile). Among adults, 52.3 percent of African American and 50.1 percent of Mexican American women were overweight, compared to 33.5 percent of white women. In the first two groups, the prevalence of obesity is even higher in women 40–69 years old; it is about 55–60 percent. African American and Mexican American women are at greatly increased risk of being obese and of having health complications associated with obesity. Indeed, the prevalence of high blood pressure and the death rates due to heart disease, stroke, and adult-onset diabetes are about twice as great in black women as in white women of similar age.

This raises the question of whether African American and Mexican American children and adolescents should receive special attention in obesity prevention (Melnyk et al. 1994). From an ethical standpoint, one may rightly question whether a specific group of people should be singled out for any reason. Why not just hope that the group at high risk gets the same message as everybody else? Few people would argue with the premise that unfair intrusion and discrimination should never occur when health interventions are targeted toward any one group. But rather than assuming that discrimination is inevitable in such an intervention, let's ask this question: "Is it fair for individuals at very high risk of developing a condition which can cause disease *not* to receive special attention that might prevent it?"

Consider the case of genetic screening for sickle cell disease. African Americans are far more likely than others to have this disease, which now can be diagnosed at birth. Preventive treatment, including daily penicillin, is effective in preventing death in childhood. Most states have screening programs to find this disease, not only in African American children but also in those of Mediterranean descent and in Asians. As a result, thousands of lives have been saved. There are many other examples of ways in which society has benefitted from interventions targeting high-risk groups. Educational interventions which are sensitive to the culture and social traditions of the target population may be very effective.

A second issue related to such interventions is whether the targeted population possesses any characteristics that make obesity more likely than in another population. This is not an easy question to answer, since generalizations about people's physiology or biochemistry based on skin color are very difficult to prove. I have cited evidence in chapter 5 that racial differences in rates of energy expenditure may eventually explain differences in rates of overweight and obesity.

Let's limit our discussion to black female adolescents, although we know that other groups of children and adolescents, such as Native Americans, U. S.-born Hmong, Puerto Ricans, and Hawaiians and other Pacific Islanders, are also at high risk for obesity. The following examples may provide insight into the risks and benefits of obesity prevention among African American girls:

1. By adolescence, more black girls than whites tend to be heavy. This does not appear to be due to differences in educational level. The NHLBI Growth and Health Study (Kimm

et al. 1996) has reported that among 9- and 10-year-old girls, white girls living in families with high levels of parent education and income were less obese than white girls whose parents had lower income and education levels. However, obesity among black girls in this study appeared to be independent of family income and education.

2. At least one study (Kumanyika et al. 1993) has suggested that black women may be less preoccupied with dieting and are generally more tolerant of overweight than other groups. These investigators found that, of the overweight black women interviewed who acknowledged that they were overweight, 40 percent considered their figures to be "attractive."

3. Using data from the NHLBI Growth and Health Study, Suzanne McNutt and collaborators compared eating practices of 9- and 10-year-old black girls (McNutt et al. 1997). They discovered that black girls were more likely than white girls to practice eating behaviors that are associated with weight gain, such as eating while doing homework, eating big helpings of food, sneaking food, and buying snack food.

4. Again using data from the NHLBI Growth and Health Study, George Schreiber and coworkers reported that 40 percent of 9- and 10-year-old black girls and white girls were trying to lose weight, and that there were no significant differences between black girls and white girls trying to do so (Schreiber et al. 1996). However, significantly more black girls than white girls were trying to *gain* weight. An important predictor in their doing so was their mothers telling them that they were too thin.

In summary, if preventive interventions are to be carried out among particular groups of people at high risk for obesity, close attention must be paid to the cultural and social characteristics of those groups, whether they are African American, Mexican American, or other. What this means is that a great deal more effort is necessary on the part of interventionists than simply providing generic prevention information designed for the general public.

Summary

We have learned in this chapter that the calorie and fat intake of children and adolescents has increased in recent years, and that physical activity levels have decreased. We have also enumerated some of the constraints faced by schools in implementing school health curricula, including obesity-prevention strategies, such as those shown to be effective in the CATCH demonstration. We have brought attention to a few of the federal and state programs designed to foster healthy eating and physical activity practices among Americans, and have discussed the challenges faced by parents who want to do all they can to prevent their children from becoming obese. Finally, we have discussed the possibility of targeting groups at high risk for obesity, noting that sensitivity would need to be part of any such action.

7. If Prevention Doesn't Work

All those who drink of this remedy recover in a short time, except those whom it does not help, who die. Therefore, it is obvious that it fails only in incurable cases.

Galen

If obesity is increasing to the extent that is described in chapter 2, we can conclude that efforts at prevention haven't worked very well in America, at least since the 1960s. Statistics reveal that in 1989–90, about 44 million Americans aged 18 years or older were trying to lose weight—38 percent of adult women and 24 percent of adult men (Horm et al. 1993). Young people also have been concerned with their weight: during this same time period, an estimated 44 percent of high school girls and 15 percent of boys reported that they were trying to lose weight. Another 26 percent of girls and 15 percent of boys said they were trying to avoid gaining weight (Serdula et al. 1993). Even preadolescent girls think about weight control: 40 percent of the 9- and 10-year-old girls in the NHLBI Growth and Health Study reported that they were trying to lose weight (Schreiber et al. 1996).

How do people try to lose weight? The majority (80 percent) of adults try to do so by eating less than usual and 60 percent by increasing physical activity. A much smaller proportion do both. Some attempt weight control by refraining from eating before bedtime. Adolescents most commonly try to lose weight by increasing exercise and skipping meals. Only a minority say they do so by using "diet pills" or by inducing vomiting after eating (Serdula et al. 1993).

Why do people want to lose weight? Reasons most often given are improvement of self-image and sexual attractiveness and concern about the health consequences of being overweight and about the social discrimination that some obese people have to live with. Adolescence can be a tough time for anyone, especially for an obese child who wants to be included in the group, not thought of as "different." Parents of smaller children worry about their youngsters being teased or suffering from social rejection and about their own difficulties in finding clothes that will fit an obese child.

When obese adults or parents of obese children realize that previous weight control efforts have been unsuccessful, they may try out self-instruction books and videotapes, commercial dietary products, or exercise devices. Some may turn to physicians, psychologists, dietitians, exercise physiologists, and other health professionals for help. Many people are understandably confused about which programs or products are safe, reliable, and effective. Because the demand for information about weight loss has been so great, and since Americans spend over $30 billion a year in weight loss efforts, the National Institutes of Health convened a national conference in 1992 to help people make intelligent decisions about weight control programs and products. In spite of the availability of this information (National Institutes of Health Technology Assessment Conference Panel 1992), many people seem to be either unwilling or unable to spend the time required to get the necessary information so that they can make rational choices. They may be looking for a quick fix. And when they discover that long-term weight control may only be attainable by constant, lifelong attention to diet and exercise habits, and not through a product that "burns fat off while you sleep," they become discouraged and abandon further attempts at control.

Very little information is available on successful weight control strategies for children, because we are in the early stages of knowing exactly how to successfully treat obesity in this age group. Treatment of an obese child is more difficult than treatment of an obese adult for several reasons: because obesity is harder to diagnose in children, because treatment has to be negotiated through parents, grandparents, school cafeteria managers, and others, and because great care must be taken in trying to help a child control weight at a time in life when natural growth requirements generally result in a weight increase. (Children are in no way "little adults," since they are progressing through various stages of physical, neurologic, and social development.) Until we have more experience, we have to use some of the information gathered from treatment of obese adults in the treatment of obese children.

Treatment of obesity has been based on several models. One is the *moral model*, which teaches the individual to accept that he or she is helpless to correct a certain problem without recognizing and depending on a "higher power," as well as on lifetime group support. Alcoholics Anonymous is an example of this model. Another is the *self-control model*, which assumes that an individual has become obese because he or she failed to learn about healthy diet and exercise practices earlier in life. Treatment consists of reeducating the obese individual and helping change behaviors that probably led to the obesity. A third is the *medical model*, which assumes that obesity is a disease arising from faulty physiologic or biochemical processes, and is best managed by hospitalization, drugs to decrease appetite or increase metabolic rate, and procedures such as surgery or wiring the mouth partially shut to decrease food absorption, intake, or both.

The *food dependency model* contains elements of both the moral and the medical models. It is based on the idea that the obese person has become dependent on food, as another person might become dependent on alcohol or drugs, and treatment is directed toward decreasing this dependency.

Finally, the *continuous care and problem-solving model*, developed by Dr. Michael Perri at the University of Florida and his colleagues, is based on the belief that obesity is a chronic, lifelong condition that in many people requires continuous and indefinite assistance from a qualified therapist. Therapy is based on identifying the unique conditions in a person's life that led to obesity—such as family structure and dynamics, learning ability, school or work requirements, eating and physical activity behaviors—and then devising a plan of action to solve those problems (Perri et al. 1992).

The success of an adult therapeutic program depends on how prepared and willing the obese person is to undergo treatment. Dr. James Prochaska and his colleagues at the University of Rhode Island, as well as other investigators, have helped us to better understand the psychology of changes in human behavior by introducing a *stages of change* model (Prochaska et al. 1992). This model can be applied to treatment of smoking, alcoholism, obesity, or other conditions: people in the "precontemplation" stage who have never considered losing weight are unlikely to respond to even the best treatment program. Those in the "contemplation" stage are aware of a problem and have thought about correcting it, but are as yet uncommitted to action. People in the "decision-making" stage (those who say they are determined to lose weight), and others in the "active change" stage (those who are already making the changes necessary to lose weight) are much more likely to respond to treatment efforts. Therapeutic plans would seem to have the highest chance of success if they fit the obese individual's level of preparedness for change. Of course, there is little information about the effectiveness of evaluating the stages of change as part of a therapeutic program for obese children.

Nutrition Education

The foundation of weight control programs for children is the child's and the family's knowledge of which foods are most likely to cause or maintain obesity. Since parents bear the responsibility for buying and preparing foods, they must always be included in nutrition education efforts. Basic nutrition education is usually performed by dietitians, who are experts in teaching the basic food groups, kcal requirements at various ages, and requirements for minerals such as iron, calcium, and sodium, and for other nutrients. Counselling by dietitians generally follows the *Dietary Guidelines for Americans* (see chapter 6), and emphasizes the recommendation that total dietary fat be limited to 30 percent of total kcals, saturated fat to 10 percent of total kcals, and cholesterol to 300 mg/day. In recent years, dietitians have led the effort to encourage families to follow the *5-a-day rule*: 5 servings each day of any combination of vegetables and fruits, which not only supply the right mix of calories, vitamins, and minerals but also displace more calorie-dense foods from the diet.

The nutrition education programs for obese children used by many dietitians may be based on the *exchange system* of the American Dietetic and the American Diabetic Associations, in which food equivalents are stressed. In this system, foods are grouped into 6 basic categories (starch, meat, vegetable, fruit, milk, and fat), and exchanges within each group can be selected based on macronutrient and kcal content. For example, one exchange from the starch list contains 80 kcals, derived from 20 grams of carbohydrate. An ounce of bread or one-half cup of cereal or corn represents one starch exchange. The number of exchanges per group required to attain a certain caloric intake is provided in tables, so that an individual can select among many various foods. Although this system may be useful for those who have the time and resolve to use it, I have not found it to be practical for parents of obese children.

A closely related system, the *stoplight diet*, has been developed by Dr. Leonard Epstein and his associates (Epstein 1988). In this system, foods are grouped into 1 of 3 color sections (red, yellow, and green) depending on their fat content. Most children readily understand the analogy to a traffic light. "Red" foods are those which make us gain weight, such as fried foods, sausages, french fried potatoes, jumbo hamburgers, and pizza with pepperoni topping. "Green" foods are those that we may eat freely: broccoli, asparagus, dill pickles, cabbage, beets—almost any food that is in the produce section of a supermarket. "Yellow" foods require caution, but generally should be eaten in limited amounts: corn, beans, pasta, breads, and cereals. Most families can understand this excellent system, and we have found it to be indispensable in our clinics.

Calorie Restriction Diets

The obese child presents a special challenge for any dietary intervention because of nutritional requirements for normal growth. Inappropriate restriction of food can be detrimental to the growth process, resulting in stunting or other evidence of nutritional deprivation. For this reason, diets which severely restrict kcal intake are generally reserved for the most severely obese children, and should be carried out under the direction or with the assistance of a physician who has experience with such diets. Two of these are effective for short-term weight loss: the *very low kcal diet* (*VLCD*), and the *protein-sparing modified fast diet* (*PSMF*). Both are alternatives to fasting, and neither should be used for long-term weight maintenance. In the 1970s, VLCD diets (usually 800 liquid kcals/day) were associated with several adult deaths in this country; these were thought to be due to poor-quality protein in the dietary preparations. Today, even with the use of high-quality protein in VLCD formulas, muscle wasting, osteoporosis (thinning of the bones), and gallstone formation can occur, depending upon the duration of the diet and the quality of follow-up medical care. VLCDs should not be used in children with kidney or liver disease, diabetes, or chronic infections (National Task Force on the Prevention and Treatment of Obesity 1993).

The protein-sparing modified fast diet (Bistrian 1978) is similar to the VLCD, except that it consists of solid food. It typically contains about 800 kcal per day, and consists of approximately

2 grams per kilogram ideal body weight of animal protein (such as broiled lean beef or skinless chicken, water-packed tuna, boiled shrimp), and low-carbohydrate vegetables (such as broccoli, beets, squash, carrots, cauliflower, and cabbage). Its use requires vitamin, calcium, and potassium supplementation, and at least 2 liters of water or other calorie-free liquids a day. Inclusion of high-quality protein helps preserve muscle mass, but, as with VLCDs, the use of this diet carries a risk of gallstones, kidney stones, and dehydration. Children can expect to lose about 2 pounds a week; this diet should never be used on a long-term basis.

Increasing Physical Activity

In chapter 5 we learned that when people reduce their energy intake, their resting metabolic rates also decrease, making it more difficult to lose weight. This phenomenon generally protects us when food is scarce. On the other hand, exercise does not lead to a decrease in resting metabolic rate, but can result in significant expenditure of energy. This is why the first two components of successful weight control programs, diet modification and exercise, must go hand in hand.

There are very few systems of practical exercise recommendations for obese children. Therapists do not generally refer children to exercise physiologists or recreation therapists for planning daily exercise programs, depending instead on parents and caretakers to allow preschool children to follow their natural instincts for physical movement, and helping school-age children and adolescents get involved in group activities. The challenge for the health professional trying to prevent obesity or to assist the obese child and his or her family is to design a program of daily exercise that will be at a comfortable level and that can be carried out for the rest of the child's life.

This does not mean that every child must become a soccer or basketball player, or a world-class swimmer, although these are excellent activities. One of the best programs for young children is the one promulgated by Rae Pica, which teaches natural movement coupled with music (Pica 1995). Extended walking (20–30 minutes or more) is perhaps the best example of a simple exercise in which children from kindergarten through high school can participate with their parents. Family members can use this time not only for the expenditure of energy but for talking with each other. Exercise strategies for children in urban rather than rural settings, for those with disabilities, or for those living in unsafe neighborhoods may require a great deal of creative thinking by the therapist and the family. In any case, every obese child needs to have an exercise program which is tailored to his or her capabilities and living circumstances.

Behavior Modification

An indispensable component of a basic weight control program for children involves correcting some of the habits acquired earlier in life which promoted obesity and teaching the child to react appropriately to the everyday circumstances which increase the risk of obesity. This is known as behavior modification (Perri et al. 1992), and its success depends on the willingness of the parents to participate.

One technique of behavior modification commonly used is *self-monitoring*, which usually takes the form of a dietary and exercise diary in which the kind and amount of every food and physical activity is recorded, and is then reviewed by the therapist at each visit. Self-monitoring is useful for focusing on what foods are usually being consumed. However, most families tire of keeping a logbook up to date after the first few weeks, and the responsibility can become a chore rather than a learning experience.

A second technique is *stimulus (cue) control*, which simply means trying to remove or minimize the factors in children's environments which make them think of eating. There are many ways parents can do this: by restricting eating to the kitchen or dining room, by refraining from bringing calorie-dense food into the home, by cooking only enough food for one serving, by serving their children's plates, by finding ways to eat slowly (such as putting utensils down between bites), and by eliminating distractions such as television which promote rapid and excessive eating. In the best strategies parents do not prompt children to clean their plates but encourage them always to leave a little. Parents may have difficulty with some of these practices because of negative reactions by other household members, especially those without weight problems. It is therefore critically important to emphasize from the beginning the importance of healthy eating for all family members, not just the one who is obese.

A third technique used to modify obesity-promoting behavior is called *cognitive restructuring*. This is just a lofty way of saying "attitude change." Parents know that obese kids become upset when someone calls attention to their weight, and may consider themselves failures. Then, to feel better, they may overeat, which makes the situation worse. Cognitive restructuring helps kids learn to anticipate and deal with the teasing, criticism, or thoughtless comments of others, and in doing so to minimize their own disappointment with themselves.

Here's how cognitive restructuring works: children are presented with hypothetical situations which they are likely to encounter, and taught to plan their responses in advance. For example, if a child is attempting weight control but spends money earned on a cheeseburger, fried potatoes, and a milkshake, he or she may say, "I'm a failure. I'll never be able to do what I know is good for me, and I'll never lose weight." Such a child may experience guilt or even depression, and may eat even more to feel better. Cognitive restructuring would teach the child to say something like this: "I promised myself that I would try to keep my weight constant, and this won't help me do that. But just because I made this mistake, I'm not going to give up on myself. What can I do in the future to make sure this doesn't happen again?" The reader can see that cognitive restructuring is generally reserved for older children and adults. In any case, the success of this technique depends on the parents' unequivocal support.

Many therapists advocate tangible rewards to help reinforce desirable behavior changes. Reasonable, well-planned, nonfood rewards can give the child a sense of accomplishment and self-worth. Weight loss is often sufficient reward for many young people, enabling them, for example, to wear the same kinds of clothes their friends are wearing. Some therapeutic programs use a "contract" by which parents, at the beginning of therapy, deposit money that is returned gradually each time the child attends a session, loses weight, or achieves another prearranged objective.

In discussing each of the above three categories, I have referred to the desirability and importance of family support for the obese child undergoing therapy. This is not simply an opinion. At least one excellent study has demonstrated that obese children lose more weight for a longer period of time if their parents participate in the therapy (Epstein et al. 1990). There are few studies of this kind which so clearly and convincingly indicate the importance of the family, especially the parents, taking part in an obese child's effort to achieve weight control.

Length of Treatment for the Obese Child

There is also little objective information available on the optimal length of time that children should remain in therapy for obesity. In our Pediatric Preventive Cardiology Clinics at the University of Mississippi, we approach the problem of obesity as a life-long condition, just as we do diabetes, sickle cell anemia, and other chronic diseases. Since we do not know beforehand which obese children will or will not become obese adults, we ask that families entering our treatment program be prepared to attend clinic every one to three months, depending on their location and transportation circumstances. Our experience has been that many families may require only two or three visits before the obese child shows a pattern of weight control and can safely be followed at intervals of three to four months. Others may require shorter intervals. Our practice is to encourage children and their families to return to our clinics indefinitely for reinforcement.

How Do You Spell "Success"?

There are several standards by which weight loss or control can be measured. These include long-term weight loss to a desirable level, progress in achieving an ideal body weight or an ideal body mass index, decreases in estimates of body fat determined by underwater weighing or computerized tomography (the CAT scan), and improvement in existing complications of obesity (such as lower blood pressure readings, lower blood glucose levels, improvement of symptoms of obstructive sleep apnea, and relief of depression).

Defining how much weight, if any, children should lose is very important, since most are experiencing normal daily growth in height and muscle mass and therefore should be expected to gain some weight. As I have pointed out earlier, weight loss may actually be detrimental to a growing child's health. The challenge to the therapist is to design a weight control strategy which on the one hand helps the child meet the energy demands of normal growth, yet on the other hand achieves some measure of progress.

Nothing is as discouraging to everyone involved as when the obese child closely follows dietary and exercise recommendations, and yet on follow-up visits shows no demonstrable weight loss or maybe even small gains. For this reason, we measure success in our clinics by comparing changes in body mass index (Smith et al. 1997), percent overweight, and triceps skinfold measurement, as well as by assessing favorable changes in self-image and corrections in family, school, and other environmental influences which may have contributed to obesity. We believe that these measures are specific to each child. Let's use a true case report as an example:

> LC, accompanied by her mother and paternal grandmother, first visited our clinic when she was almost 8 years old. Her weight was 63.7 kg (140 pounds), and her height was 137 cm (nearly 54 inches). Her body mass index was 33.9 (upper limit of normal for her age was 21.0); her weight was approximately 77 percent greater than her estimated ideal weight for height. Her triceps skinfold measurement was 42 mm (upper limit of normal was 22 mm). Blood pressure measurements averaged 122/52; normal blood pressure for her age, sex, and height was 112/72.
>
> Of particular concern was the fact that LC and her family lived next door to the paternal grandmother, who was the dominating influence in their family. She showered LC with attention by buying her clothes and toys and by frequently taking her out to eat at fast food hamburger locations. She also instructed LC's mother about the "best" foods for LC: traditional southern foods high in fat and kcals, such as fried chicken, rice and gravy, and casserole dishes. LC's parents wanted her to gain control of her weight, but were also dependent on the grandmother for child care, since they both worked and were financially stressed. Although LC lost about 4 pounds in the 2 months after her first visit, she did not return to clinic for the next year and a half. When she did return, her mother told us that she had finally realized that the grandmother's influence, though well intentioned, had become detrimental to LC's health, and she now forbade LC to spend time with her grandmother unless she or LC's father accompanied her. The family had begun to practice nutrition and exercise habits which we had recommended, and which caused significant distress to the grandmother.
>
> At her last visit, LC's weight was 69 kg (152 pounds) and her height was 148.1 cm (58.3 inches). Her body mass index had therefore decreased to 31.4 because of her increased height, and

her weight had now decreased to approximately 53 percent over her ideal weight for current height. Triceps skinfold measurement had decreased from 42 to 33 mm. Blood pressure was 106/70, well within normal range for that height.

LC's mother later said that things were "getting better" with her mother-in-law since everyone in the family now understood that LC's parents were in charge of raising their own child.

Using weight alone as a measure of success in this child would have led to a conclusion of failure, since her weight actually increased by 12 pounds over about 18 months. When weight gain due to normal linear (height) growth was factored in, LC was still overweight for her height, but decreases in body mass index and ideal weight for height showed marked improvement. The decrease in triceps skinfold measurement demonstrated that the decrease in body mass index was most likely due to a decrease in body fat content, not in lean body mass. And just as important from the perspective of long-term change in LC's case is the fact that her parents assumed their rightful places as nurturers, accepting responsibility for her nutritional, recreational, emotional, and spiritual direction.

Pharmacologic Therapy for Obesity

In 1996 and 1997, reports were published of serious heart and lung disease in humans (Abenhaim et al. 1996; Connolly et al. 1997) and long-lasting toxic changes in brains of experimental animals associated with fenfluramine (McCann 1997), a drug used to treat obesity in adults. In 1997, the Food and Drug Administration (FDA) withdrew approval of fenfluramine (Pondimin), as well as dexfenfluramine (Redux) because of increasing concerns about adverse side effects. This new information, coupled with the longer-standing controversy about whether medications to control appetite should be used under any except the most desperate circumstances, has forced all therapists to reevaluate the safety and effectiveness of these drugs.

Compared to adults, obese children and adolescents have rarely used drug therapy, because few scientific studies regarding this age group show these drugs to be effective in obese children. Most antiobesity drugs are limited by manufacturers to use in individuals above the age of 12 years.

Amphetamines, the first class of drugs used to treat obesity in American adults, decreased the desire for food in many who used them. However, this class of drugs was quickly discovered to have the potential for addiction, mainly because taking them resulted in a sense of well-being. Subsequently, use of "diet pills" became tightly regulated by boards of medical licensure in most states. Because of this, and because of the FDA requirement of evidence of their effectiveness, the development of other antiobesity drugs has been a slow and tedious process. Moreover, use of these drugs is recommended only for up to one year. Since lost weight is nearly always regained when use is discontinued, the effectiveness of these drugs may depend upon the obese individual continuing to take them for many months or even years. For all of these reasons, the 1996 report of the National Task Force on the Prevention and Treatment of Obesity concluded that "pharmacotherapy cannot be recommended for routine use in obese individuals, although it may be helpful in carefully selected patients" (Anonymous 1996).

Use of antiobesity drugs has also been controversial because some physicians who have prescribed them have not tied their use to helping patients change poor nutrition and exercise habits. In most busy clinics, it is a lot easier for a physician to write a prescription for a drug and go on to the next patient than it is to engage in an hour-long counselling session in an effort to determine some of the factors that caused the person's obesity in the first place.

With the above caveat, I will briefly describe some of the drugs that have been used commonly in adults, so that parents and others will be aware of their names and the different ways in which they act.

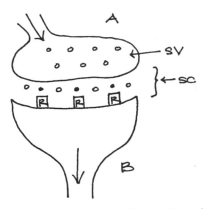

FIG. 7.1. The chemical transmission of an electrical impulse (first arrow) travelling along nerve fiber A. The impulse stimulates release of a neurotransmitter, such as norepinephrine or serotonin stored in packets called synaptic vesicles (SV), into the space called the synaptic cleft (SC) between nerve fibers A and B. The neurotransmitter combines with specific receptors (R) on the cell membrane of nerve fiber B, altering its electrical charge, and the impulse continues along nerve fiber B. The neurotransmitter is then taken up by nerve fiber A again to be stored in synaptic vesicles, unless a drug prevents it from doing so.

How Antiobesity Drugs Work

Antiobesity drugs have their effect either centrally (in the central nervous system) or peripherally (at some location outside the central nervous system.) *Centrally acting drugs* work by interfering with the complex chemical processes in the brain responsible for appetite or satiety.

To understand this better, let's review briefly how electrical impulses are transmitted between nerve cells in the brain by looking at figure 7.1. Imagine that an electrical impulse is travelling along brain nerve fiber A. It eventually reaches brain nerve fiber B. How does this impulse get across the space from nerve A to nerve B? Easy. The impulse in nerve fiber A causes tiny packets of a chemical to be released into the space between the two nerve fibers. This chemical, called a neurotransmitter, then combines for a short time with specific receptors on nerve fiber B's cell membrane. This combination changes the electrical charge on nerve fiber B's cell membrane, allowing the impulse to be transmitted from nerve fiber A to nerve fiber B in a very short time. The neurotransmitter is then taken up again by nerve fiber A (a process known as "reuptake"), ready for another impulse to be transmitted.

Several different chemicals in the brain transmit nerve impulses. The two groups which have been studied the most in appetite control are catecholamines and serotonin. (We learned a little about the catecholamines epinephrine and norepinephrine in chapter 5.) Drugs which act either by stimulating the release of a catecholamine into the space between nerve fibers or which mimic the actions of catecholamines are called catecholaminergic drugs. Examples of catecholaminergic drugs which act as central nervous system stimulants to decrease appetite are diethylpropion (Tenuate), phentermine (Phentride), mazindol (Sanorex), and phenylpropanolamine (Dexatrim). Amphetamine is an example of a drug that acts in both ways described above.

Serotoninergic drugs act differently from catecholaminergic drugs. They appear to increase and extend the sense of satiety and well-being after food is eaten, rather than suppressing appetite as a result of stimulation of the central nervous system. In other words, hunger is often postponed when these drugs are taken. Dexfenfluramine (Redux) both inhibits the reuptake of serotonin and causes an increased release of serotonin from the nerve cell. Sibutramine (Meridia), approved for human use in late 1997, acts by inhibiting reuptake of the neurotransmitters serotonin and norepinephrine. Used to treat depression, *dl*-fluoxetine (Prozac) also inhibits reuptake of serotonin, and helps control appetite in about 20-30 percent of those taking it for treatment of obesity. The well-known "phen-fen" combination is the combination of two drugs, phentermine and *dl*-fenfluramine.

Peripherally acting drugs are those which alter reactions of organs. One example is ephedrine, which is a centrally acting drug, but one that also affects the sympathetic nervous system. It increases the heart rate and blood pressure, and helps relax the smooth muscles in the bronchial tree; it has therefore been used in the treatment of asthma. Its side effects have made it a poor drug for long-term weight loss. A second example is thyroid hormone, which may increase the resting metabolic rate, but in so doing induces loss of muscle mass.

In summary, pharmacological treatment of obesity in children and adolescents is not a generally acceptable option at the present time, because more studies are needed to demonstrate the effectiveness and the safety of these drugs in this age group.

Aggressive Therapy for Severe Childhood Obesity: Dental Wiring, Surgery, and Alternative Living Environments

Tragically, a few children are severely obese when they enter treatment programs. They and their families may have tried unsuccessfully many times to change diet and exercise habits. Reasons for failure may include lack of interest by parents and other family members or disabilities in the child which make learning good nutrition practices or engaging in physical activity impossible. Some of these children have developed complications of obesity, such as obstructive sleep apnea, pulmonary hypertension, and heart failure, as explained in chapter 1. They may have experienced life-threatening illnesses because of obesity, and without weight loss are likely to die at an early age. For them, repeated use of the techniques described above may be useless.

There are two options available for these children: physical restriction of food intake and long-term residential care. Food intake may be restricted by the temporary placement of wires on the teeth, much like braces, which nearly close the mouth and allow only liquids and small bites of food to be eaten. Even with dental wiring, it is possible for someone to consume large amounts of high-calorie, high-fat blended foods, which can defeat the purpose of the procedure. Also, for children who do have obstructive sleep apnea or pulmonary hypertension, dental wiring may be life threatening if the air passages are restricted in any way. This method of treatment is rarely used today.

A more frequently used method (Kral 1992) of restricting food intake involves the surgical placement of staples to create a small pouch in the upper part of the stomach (fig. 7.2). This procedure can be thought of as the creation of two stomachs which connect with each other: a small stomach which has a very limited capacity for food, and a larger stomach which partially digests food in a normal manner. Food enters and fills the small pouch, and the stomach signals the brain that it is full. Further food intake slows down temporarily. But after food passes from the small pouch to the larger stomach, more may be eaten.

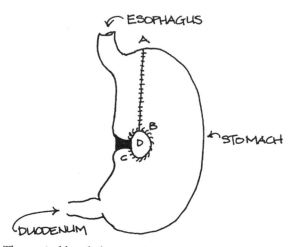

FIG. 7.2. The vertical banded gastroplasty. A row of staples is placed along the stomach between points A and B, and a band is placed at point C to create a small channel so that food can leave the stomach. A small defect (D) must be created in the stomach to allow placement of the band. The stomach is thus divided into a small upper pouch and a larger lower pouch. Food entering the lower pouch begins to be digested in a normal manner by the stomach.

This operation has helped many people, including adolescents and some children. Unfortunately, the small pouch can stretch or the staples can come out if excessive amounts of food are eaten, so that the small stomach can become large, and the effects of the operation are lost. Many people overconsume high-fat, high-kcal liquids after this operation and suffer from vomiting because of insufficient chewing or excessive intake of liquids after eating. In addition, iron and other deficiencies can occur.

A second surgical procedure consists of creating a small upper stomach pouch which does not communicate with the rest of the stomach, but which instead empties directly into the small intestine. The effect—a feeling of fullness—is the same as that produced by the other operation, but if the individual overeats or overdrinks, excessive food or liquid is dumped directly into the intestine, causing indigestion and diarrhea. Thus, the individual quickly learns to eat modestly after this operation. Since iron, vitamin B-12, and other deficiencies can occur with this procedure, its use requires continuous and careful long-term follow-up.

Surgical treatment of obesity should be implemented only when intensive attempts to modify behavior have been unsuccessful, or when children have experienced life-threatening complications of obesity. Morbidly obese people frequently develop complications from being anesthetized, and the excessive fat tissue on their abdomens can be very slow to heal or can become infected after surgery. Many centers report encouraging results with these surgical procedures, which can be life-saving for children and adolescents.

Many obese children live in families in which changes in eating and exercise habits are very improbable. Although the parents may be loving, well educated, and knowledgeable, they find it impossible to change the longstanding habits which caused the obesity. Other obese children live in homes in which they receive inadequate attention: their parents or caretakers may be physically or mentally ill; their parents may have abandoned them so that they are in the care of a grandparent; a large number of extended family members may live in the home; or adult caretakers may have their hands full with two jobs or another family member who is severely disabled. Still other children have psychiatric conditions, such as serious depression, or developmental conditions, including mental retardation, which make it unlikely that they or their families will ever be able to implement necessary life changes to ameliorate obesity.

In any of these situations, repeated and prolonged attempts at behavior modification may have been unsuccessful, and the negative reaction of family members to new foods or new ways of preparing food may precipitate family stress. The obese child may be singled out for hostile attention, or may simply overeat in an effort to feel better. We often see children in our clinics who live in chaotic home circumstances and, while there may not be outright abuse or neglect, faulty family dynamics or adverse living circumstances have clearly contributed to their obesity. Dramatic changes in their living circumstances, including outplacement in a foster or group home, may be necessary to effect any long-lasting behavior modification. The following example illustrates how living circumstances or family dynamics can contribute to obesity:

> SG was 12 years old when he was first seen in our clinic, and weighed 184 pounds, which was 184 percent of his ideal weight for height. His maternal grandmother was his legal guardian. He ate high-fat breakfasts at home, and his school regularly served high-fat lunches, including pizza, corn dogs, hamburgers and french fries, and fried chicken with rice and gravy. His grandmother served the same kind of foods for supper and on weekends. She said that it would be hard to change anything because of her husband's tastes. SG spent a summer in another state with an aunt who insisted on regular exercise and a healthy diet for her children and for SG. When he returned home after 2 months, SG had lost 18 pounds. Nine months after returning to his usual environment, he weighed 4 pounds more than at his first visit.

We see many children in our clinics whose living circumstances not only promote obesity but also threaten their normal development as human beings. Although we have recommended and assisted in placing severely obese children outside their homes for lengthy periods, we do so with the knowledge that there is little scientific information on whether such care effects substantial behavioral change (Boeck et al. 1993).

The Treatment Program for Obese Children and Adolescents at the University of Mississippi Medical Center

So that the reader can gain better insight into how one obesity treatment program works, I have provided the following summary of the philosophy and operation of our own clinic. It is not unique. We have built our program on the experience of many others.

1. We try never to do harm to an obese child or the family. We try to avoid complicating the difficulties of obesity by contributing to other problems such as anorexia, bulimia, and family discord. We think that there are conditions worse than obesity.

2. We also believe that, until proven otherwise, obesity can be a lifelong condition that may result in premature death or disability for many adults, and that there is no good way to determine a priori which obese child or adolescent will become an obese adult (see chapter 2). Consequently, we believe in frequently repeated education efforts directed at the child and the family. We seek long-term rather than short-term results.

3. We think that the first step in weight loss is weight control. We believe that what is crucial to a child is his or her normal, healthy development as a human being, and that includes appropriate dietary and exercise practices.

4. We believe that successful weight management for most children depends upon interested, supportive parents and other family members.

5. We try to discover the unique circumstances that were likely to have led to obesity, including details of a child's daily life in home, school, and work environments, and to base our therapeutic recommendations on modifying those circumstances when possible. For this task, we often call upon the expertise of a professional family therapist. We also try to imagine how we would implement the treatment objectives that we recommend to families, taking into account their unique economic and social challenges.

6. We keep in mind that obese children may encounter cruel and unthinking remarks from many people, and we attempt to help them find ways in which they can react positively, rather than negatively, to such insensitivity.

7. We accept any child into our clinic, including those with disabilities.

When an obese child is referred to our clinic, we ask that both parents or guardians come in also, so that we can obtain the child's family and personal medical history and learn about the family configuration. In addition to learning about eating patterns, which help us determine whether a child is a "grazer" or a binge eater, we look for overly protective relationships between the parent and child which may have occurred because of prior illnesses. We search for disabling health conditions, such as asthma, which might limit a child's physical activity or require use of drugs (for example, prednisone) that stimulate appetite and lead to obesity, or other conditions, such as spinal defects, which limit physical activity and cause less energy than usual to be expended (Smith et al. 1999). We define a child's physical sexual maturity rating, including a girl's menstrual history, since regularly occurring menstrual periods make it unlikely that she has the polycystic ovary disease, which can be both a cause and an effect of obesity. Boys having small testicles and retardation may be at especially high risk for obesity.[12] Physical examination of the obese child may also reveal any of the consequences of obesity mentioned in chapter 1.

In our clinics, we do little laboratory testing.[13] Families often want to attribute a child's obesity to "a gland problem," but unfortunately this is seldom the cause. Insufficient thyroid hormone (hypothyroidism) is a rare cause of obesity in children, but those with this condition may have weight gain because of water retention. Obesity is seldom a prominent feature of children with hypothyroidism. The medical literature contains little evidence of the effectiveness of thyroid supplementation in the treatment of obesity. In addition, few obese children have diseases of the adrenal glands, in which abnormal amounts of critically important hormones, such as cortisol, are secreted.

In summary, we have found that the family and medical history, along with a thorough physical examination by a pediatrician or other primary practitioner who has experience with obese children and adolescents, is a necessary prerequisite for formulating a treatment plan. A team approach, which involves using an experienced dietitian and a psychologist attuned to the possible influence of family dynamics on a child's obesity, has been very helpful in many cases.

Summary

In this chapter we have learned that nutrition education and behavior modification involving eating and exercise are the cornerstones of obesity treatment. We have also learned that the obese child's family must be involved in the treatment, and we have been introduced to the continuous care and problem-solving model of therapy. We have seen why drug treatment of childhood obesity is not usually an option, and what the three methods of "aggressive" treatment are in cases of severe obesity. The chapter concludes with a summary of the treatment program at one medical center.

8. The Great Beyond: New Frontiers in the Treatment of Obesity

Not only do people differ metabolically from rats, they also differ quite a lot from other people.

Professor J. S. Garrow, *Obesity and Related Diseases*

Although the title of this book is *Understanding Childhood Obesity*, it is probably apparent by now that obesity is a complex condition that no one fully understands. In the previous chapters we have become acquainted with areas that hold the most promise for further research; the possible reasons for the dramatic increase of obesity in Americans over the past 35 years; the psychologic and physiologic factors surrounding food intake; how food is digested, absorbed, and assimilated into various cells of our bodies in a usable form; how energy is released by the combustion of proteins, fats, and carbohydrates, and how factors such as insulin influence energy utilization; and the ways in which we try to prevent obesity or to treat it when efforts at prevention have failed. We have learned about energy balance and how it is measured and about genetic and environmental determinants of obesity.

And yet, for each explanation offered, many new and unanswered questions appear. Fortunately, curiosity is a trait found generally in human beings and particularly in scientists. I believe that human curiosity about obesity will eventually lead us to understand more fully how and why obesity occurs, as we have learned about the causes of polio, sickle cell anemia, and AIDS. We will one day know why many of us overeat, in defiance of signals from our bodies that tell us to not do so; why so many of us find fatty foods more palatable than other kinds; why we prefer to watch television instead of playing with our kids; and why certain behaviors cause obesity in some and not in others. We will eventually understand obesity as we continue to build on the clues that have already been uncovered. The quest is an exciting one. Let's look at two areas that have been on the leading edge of obesity research: the brain and genes.

To start, let's expand on what we have learned about *feeding behavior*, a term that encompasses appetite, hunger, food seeking, and satiety. Imagine for a moment how difficult our lives would be if we did not have biologic, automatic signals that tell us when our bodies are running out of energy. Without these, we would have to develop some way to remind ourselves to eat, because if we didn't, our blood glucose levels would fall too low, our brains would quit functioning, and our lives would be threatened. A key element in understanding the process of obesity is knowing that blood glucose levels must be maintained within a narrow range. If glucose levels fall too low, we have to replenish them rapidly by eating; if the levels are too high, glucose is spilled into the urine, and potential energy is lost. Our need for glucose is a very strong *short-term* determinant of hunger, dictating the urgency with which we look for food. There are other determinants of how much and how fast we eat, such as the appearance, aroma, and palatability of the food, the surroundings in which we eat it, and our previous experience with particular foods.

When we have taken in enough food to satisfy our bodies' glucose needs, then we tend to quit eating—most of the time. We learned in chapter 3 about several short-term ways in which the gastrointestinal tract signals the brain that we have eaten enough, including the amount and composition of food which directly stimulates nerves in the walls of the small intestine to inform the brain that we have had sufficient food for our energy needs.

A *long-term* regulator of food-seeking behavior was proposed by Dr. Gordon Kennedy in 1953 and is known as the lipostatic theory (Kennedy 1953). Dr. Kennedy suggested that the amount of fat in our bodies is determined by the interaction between the hypothalamus (the highly specialized area of the brain discussed in chapter 3) and some factor or substance in equilibrium with stored fat. If true, this would mean that if we accumulate an excessive amount of body fat, then a signal is produced by our fat cells which is transmitted to our brains to inhibit appetite, and the process of acquiring food and eating it ends temporarily. Conversely, as body fat begins to disappear because of food deprivation or excessive energy expenditure, the strength of the signal becomes weaker, and our brains then stimulate us to look for and ingest food.

So our bodies may be programmed by basic metabolic mechanisms which are not under our conscious control either to acquire food or to stop eating, depending upon whether our fat stores are increasing or decreasing. What this really means is that we can survive as a species since we can depend on a continuous supply of energy at all times from our bodies, even though energy in our environments is quite variable.

Is there any evidence that a signal is produced by fat tissue, and that it is transmitted to our brains to influence eating behavior? There is, and the story of how this evidence came to be discovered begins with some very interesting mice and rats.

Let's talk a little more about a very important area of the brain, the hypothalamus. We won't worry too much about its anatomic location, except to say that it is just below the middle of the brain and just above the pituitary gland, which itself is just on the other side of the roof of your mouth. The hypothalamus has many important functions: it regulates body temperature, helps control the amount of water in the body, determines whether sensations are pleasant or painful, and helps us decide whether to stay and fight or run for our lives if we're threatened. It is also the primary area of the brain regulating the autonomic nervous system, which consists of the sympathetic and parasympathetic divisions (see note 6).

As we learned in chapter 3, the hypothalamus is a major determinant of feeding behavior: stimulation of the lateral hypothalamus increases appetite, and its destruction can cause just the opposite. Stimulation of the ventromedial nucleus of the hypothalamus decreases appetite, but damage to this area causes voracious eating.

What evidence is there that a lipostatic factor is produced by fat cells and that it stimulates brain centers? In 1959, Dr. G. R. Hervey reported that he had surgically connected the bloodstreams of two normal rats so that their circulations were "shared," a technique known as parabiosis (Hervey 1959). He then created a small injury in the ventromedial hypothalamus of one of the rats. The injured rat, as expected, began to eat voraciously, was never satiated, and became obese. What was interesting was that the other paired normal rat, whose hypothalamus was intact, lost all his appetite and soon died of starvation! Dr. Hervey hypothesized that the obese rat's increased fat mass produced a substance that was released into the bloodstream and reached the normal rat's hypothalamus, where it acted to depress the appetite. This important observation revealed the role of the hypothalamus in satiety.

Later, genetic scientists developed two different strains of obese mice: *ob/ob* and *db/db*. (Although there are other strains of obese mice, these two have been studied most intensively.) To become obese, each obese mouse in either of these strains had to inherit a defective gene (either *ob* or *db*) from each parent mouse, which simply means that the transmission is autosomal recessive[14] in nature. An affected obese mouse in either strain is hyperphagic (eats excessively), and expends less energy than normal. And both have other metabolic abnormalities: they develop non-insulin-dependent (type II) diabetes mellitus in spite of having higher than normal circulating insulin levels; they cannot increase their metabolic rates either in a cold environment or when they eat; they are often infertile; and their lean body mass (everything except fat) is decreased. In fact, they look a lot like the mouse who had a lesion placed in the ventromedial hypothalamus as discussed above, suggesting that either (1) they may lack the capacity to signal their brains that they have had enough to eat, or (2) their brains do not respond to such a signal.

In fact, in 1973 Dr. D. L. Coleman reported his remarkable investigations, in which both the *ob/ob* and the *db/db* strains were used, and which suggested that both of these possibilities were true (Coleman 1973). First, using the technique of parabiosis, he joined the circulations of *ob/ob* mice with those of normal control mice, and found that the weight of the *ob/ob* mice soon became normal! But *db/db* mice treated in the same way with normal controls showed no differences in weight. This suggested to him that *ob/ob* mice were deficient in some factor which regulated the amount of body fat, and that this factor was supplied by the normal rat. And it also suggested that even though the *db/db* mice produced this factor, it was simply ineffective in regulating body fat stores. Also interesting was the fact that both *ob/ob* and lean control mice died of starvation when joined with *db/db* mice, presumably because of the large amounts of this satiety factor produced by the *db/db* mice, which inhibited appetites of the *ob/ob* and control mice!

It was not until 1994 that Dr. Yiying Zhang and his colleagues at Rockefeller University, including Dr. Jeffrey Friedman, reported in what is now a landmark article in the journal *Nature* (Zhang 1994) that they had identified the defective gene responsible for obesity in *ob/ob* mice, and had identified the corresponding normal gene, called the *ob* gene, in fat cells both in normal mice and in humans. They showed that this gene was responsible for producing a specific protein, and suggested that the protein might be the long-sought satiety factor which regulates body fat mass. With the use of modern genetic technology, this *ob* gene was cloned (meaning that many copies were made experimentally), so that its protein could then be produced in relatively large quantities. This protein was eventually named leptin, from the Greek *leptos*, which means "thin."

The discovery of this gene caused great excitement among scientists and clinicians (Hamann et al. 1996). Perhaps at last the key was available that would unlock the mystery of why obesity develops in some human beings but not in others. Further investigations (Halaas et al. 1995) revealed that a defective, biologically inactive form of leptin was produced by the fat tissue of *ob/ob* obese mice, explaining why they became obese at an early age. When these mice were treated with injections of synthetic leptin, their appetites returned to normal, their energy expenditure increased to normal levels, their weight became normal, and their non-insulin-dependent diabetes disappeared! In *db/db* mice, investigations showed that the *ob* gene was overexpressed: abnormally high quantities of perfectly normal leptin were produced, and treatment with large quantities of synthetic leptin had absolutely no effect on these animals' obesity or other metabolic abnormalities. This again suggested that *db/db* mice became obese because they lacked a necessary receptor for leptin (Halaas et al. 1995; Campfield et al. 1995).

This is all fine in rodents, but is leptin really present in humans? If so, where does it work? What exactly does it control? And what controls leptin itself (Maffei et al. 1995)?

First, normal leptin is produced by the fat cells of normal or obese human beings, and the more body fat a person has, the more leptin is produced. There have been no reports of abnormal, biologically inactive leptin in humans, such as that found in obese *ob/ob* mice, and injection of synthetic leptin into either obese or nonobese adult humans has absolutely no effect on their body fat (Hamann et al. 1996). This suggests that obese humans behave a lot like *db/db* obese mice: leptin is produced in high quantities, but may not bind with a leptin receptor, and is thus metabolically inactive. Another way of saying this is that both *db/db* mice and obese humans are resistant to the effects of normal leptin. On the other hand, instead of a deficient receptor, perhaps leptin cannot cross from the circulation into the brain in some obese individuals because of its high molecular weight.

Where does leptin work, and what does it control? Could it possibly act in the hypothalamus, producing a feedback mechanism for appetite control? To try to answer this intriguing question, let's examine one of the neurotransmitters found throughout the brain, neuropeptide Y, or NPY. Recall from chapter 7 that a neurotransmitter is simply a chemical that enables the transfer of an electrical impulse from one nerve to another, or from a nerve to a specialized cell, such as a muscle or an endocrine gland cell. NPY is produced in particularly high quantites in the hypothalamus, and has long been suspected of playing a major role in appetite and weight control. For instance, chronic administration of NPY into the brains of experimental animals results in excessive food intake, decreased energy production, and—yes—obesity (Stanley et al. 1986). Substances such as antibodies which inhibit NPY also inhibit overfeeding, increase energy production, and result in normalization of weight. Moreover, there is evidence that hypothalamic NPY is elevated in the brains of our little friends, *ob/ob* mice. Administering synthetic leptin causes NPY levels to return to normal. Finally, injecting leptin into the brains of experimental animals receiving chronic injections of NPY causes overfeeding to return to normal. Thus, NPY might be a key element in a feedback mechanism involved in food intake, as depicted in figure 8.1 (Schwartz et al. 1997).

One problem with this scheme is that experimental animals that don't produce NPY are still able to regulate body weight and other metabolic functions, *and* they respond to synthetic leptin in a normal manner (Erickson et al. 1996)! So NPY may be only a part of the answer to our obesity riddle, not the whole one. Perhaps other, yet undiscovered brain substances, play a more important role in weight maintenance.

Is there evidence that a defective leptin receptor causes obesity in humans? A leptin receptor was identified in mice in 1995, and the gene which produces it has been cloned (Tartaglia et al. 1995). In *db/db* mice, a defective leptin receptor has been identified, as in the case of defective leptin in *ob/ob* mice. This defective protein explains not only why the normal leptin produced by obese *db/db* mice cannot exert its normal physiological action, but also why synthetic leptin administered to these animals has no effect. Intensive research is under way at this time to investigate the possible role of defective leptin receptors in some forms of human obesity, but to date no such receptor has been identified.

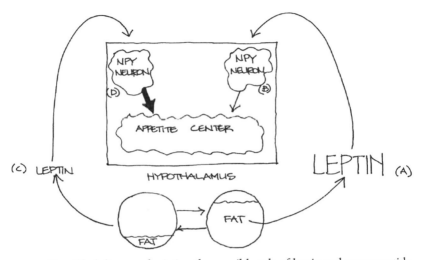

FIG. 8.I. Simplified diagram depicting the possible role of leptin and neuropeptide Y (NPY) in long-term regulation of body fat. When the fat content of a fat cell increases because of greater absorption of dietary fat, the cell's production of leptin increases (A). Leptin is transported to the hypothalamus by the bloodstream, and signals the NPY-containing brain cells to *decrease* NPY production. Since NPY is known to stimulate appetite, decreasing NPY levels reduce stimulation of the hypothalamic appetite center (B), and under normal circumstances food intake decreases. Conversely, if dietary intake of fat decreases, and the fat content of the fat cell decreases, leptin production falls (C), and production of NPY *increases* (D), enhancing the appetite and returning the fat cell to its usual state.

The Continuing Search for Answers to the Obesity Puzzle

The search for answers to the problem of obesity will continue well into the twenty-first century and perhaps beyond. It is easy for those of us who deal with obese children to say that they become obese because they are provided and eat foods excessively high in fat, or do not engage in physical activity that is sufficient to burn the energy from the food that they eat. Our genes may eventually be found to profoundly influence these two factors. We should always keep in mind the possibility that our genes control our lives to a far greater degree than we currently realize, and may explain much about why humans eat and exercise the way they do.

In chapter 5 of this book, we considered several possible ways by which obesity could develop, and examined some of the evidence that these mechanisms were under genetic control. We learned that identical twins were more likely than fraternal ones to have similar amounts of body fat, even if they were raised apart from each other. And fraternal twins were more likely to have similar amounts of body fat than were nontwin siblings. This information is a powerful argument that obesity is at least partially under genetic control, since identical twins have all genes in common, whereas fraternal twins and nontwin siblings have only some genes in common. And in chapter 7 I referred to a mutation in a gene on chromosome 15 which is closely associated with the Prader-Willi syndrome, characterized by mental retardation, excessive eating, and obesity. Currently, about 12 human obesity disorders have been linked to specific regions on chromosomes. No doubt we will eventually identify the specific genes involved and perhaps others that pertain to obesity as well.

In the meantime, we will have to depend on our knowledge of imbalances of energy intake and expenditure to explain obesity. Most of us would like to find a miracle cure or a quick fix for obesity, but this is improbable in the near future. We must rely on the time-proven remedy of reducing calories, especially fat, and engaging in regular and vigorous exercise.

Notes

1. In polycystic ovary disease, the ovary produces excessive quantities of the male hormone testosterone. Affected girls and women may have little or no menses, and may develop male-like features such as facial hair and coarse skin. About half become obese.

2. Some readers may not be familiar with the metric units "kilogram" and "centimeters" used to calculate body mass index. A kilogram is equivalent to 2.2 pounds, and a pound is equivalent to approximately 0.45 kilograms. A centimeter is equivalent to 0.39 inches, and an inch is equivalent to 2.54 centimeters.

3. Since body mass index increases as a child grows, it is somewhat more reliable as a measure when applied to adults, who have reached their maximum height. However, body mass index continues to be the measure of overweight used most often in children as well as adults.

4. The method of calculating percent body fat, given a person's body density, is as follows: we know that the density of body fat is about 0.900 gm/ml, and that the density of all other nonfat body tissues (lean body mass) is about 1.100 gm/ml. Any mixture of fat and lean tissues will result in an average body density between 0.90 gm/ml (for 100 percent fat) and 1.10 gm/ml (for 0 percent fat). Although body densities vary a little with age, sex, and race, we can say that an individual with 40 percent body fat would have an average body density of (40 percent x 0.9)+(60 percent x 1.1)=0.36+0.66=1.02 gm/ml. Another person with 10 percent body fat would have an average body density of (10 percent x 0.9)+(90 percent x 1.1)=0.09+0.99=1.08 gm/ml. Based on body densities determined experimentally by many underwater measurements on many people, we can calculate, with the help of a mathematical formula, an individual's percent body fat with an accuracy of about ± 1 percent. And knowing the percent body fat makes it possible to calculate total body fat and fat-free mass.

5. Weighing a person in air is no problem. Underwater weighing is more complex, and is usually done in a room containing a large tank of clean water the temperature of which is controlled for comfort. The individual puts on a swimsuit, inserts a snorkel into his or her mouth, and practices breathing underwater. After a scale is attached by a comfortable harness, the person enters the tank and exhales for about 5 seconds, which causes him or her to sink underwater. At this point, a weight is taken. The process is repeated about 10 times.

6. The autonomic nervous system consists of the nerves that control involuntary body functions. It is composed of the sympathetic nervous system and the parasympathetic nervous system. At each junction of an autonomic nerve and the cell it controls (such as a smooth muscle or a secretory gland), a chemical is released that transmits a nerve impulse. The chemical in the sympathetic nervous system is norepinephrine, while in the parasympathetic nervous system (and in skeletal muscle) it is acetylcholine. Both are important to digestion. Since adipose tissue is innervated by sympathetic nerve fibers, the sympathetic nervous system becomes more important in discussing the role of adipose tissue in the development of obesity (see chapters 5 and 8).

7. The term "kilocalorie," although continuing to serve us well, is gradually being replaced by the term "joule" or "kilojoule." A joule is the amount of heat generated (or expended) by an ampere of electrical current flowing through an ohm (a standard unit of electrical resistance) for 1 second. A joule is equivalent to 4.187 calories; a calorie is equivalent to 0.239 joules. A kilojoule equals 4187 calories, and a kilocalorie equals 239 kilojoules.

8. When triglycerides are broken down to glycerol and fatty acids, most of the energy released comes directly from the oxidation of the fatty acids. Remember that 3 fatty acid molecules and 1 glycerol molecule are released by the breakdown of 1 molecule of a triglyceride, the fat that is stored in adipose tissue. The glycerol is converted by the liver to glucose, which then provides 4 kcal energy per gram. But each of the 3 fatty

acids is then oxidized in a unique manner to release energy. Expressing energy in terms of ATP generated will help to underscore the differences between glucose and fat catabolism: oxidation of a molecule of glucose generates 38 molecules of ATP, while oxidation of 3 molecules of fatty acid (3 per molecule of triglyceride) generates approximately 438 molecules of ATP! Other substances in the body, such as amino acids (from protein) and lactic acid (produced by intense muscle activity) can also be transformed to glucose and used as energy.

9. Every atom has a nucleus containing positively charged particles (protons) and electrically neutral particles (neutrons). The total number of protons and neutrons determines the mass number of an atom. An atom's isotope is a nucleus which has a mass number different from another because it contains a different number of neutrons. Isotopes are chemically identical to each other. We indicate the mass number of an atom by a superscript preceding the atom and the atomic number (the number of protons) as subscript preceding the atom. The subscript following the atom tells us how many atoms of that substance are contained in the molecule. Isotopes are frequently used in medical practice and research as "tags" or "tracers" to study how a particular atom (such as carbon, hydrogen, or iodine) is metabolized by the body.

10. Complex carbohydrates are found in starchy foods such as pasta, rice, cereals, and bread and in vegetables such as potatoes. They are broken down and absorbed slowly during the digestive process, and therefore cause blood glucose levels to increase very little in the 4 hours or so after a meal. In response, relatively small amounts of insulin are secreted by the pancreas. Among its other actions, insulin inhibits hormone-sensitive lipase, the enzyme that causes stored fat to be broken down into glycerol and fatty acids. The net effect of insulin is that stored fat cannot be broken down and used as an energy source. This inhibition occurs much less with complex carbohydrates than with simple carbohydrates such as glucose, contained in, for example, candy and pastries, which can cause very high levels of insulin to be

secreted. The bottom line is that humans are more likely to *retain* fat when their diets are high in simple, refined sugars than when they eat complex carbohydrates, and the effect is probably due to the amount of insulin secreted and how fast it happens.

11. In the first year of a child's life, body fat increases because fat cells increase in size, but their number remains constant. Fat cell growth usually stabilizes after this time, although linear (height) growth continues, and children appear slimmer than when they were infants. At 4 to 7 years of age, a second period of rapid growth in body fat normally begins, in which both the size and the number of fat cells increase. The point just before this second increase in body fat is called the period of adiposity rebound. Several studies indicate that the earlier the period of adiposity rebound occurs, the greater the likelihood is that the individual will become an obese adult.

12. The Prader-Willi syndrome is characterized by mental retardation, underdeveloped sex organs, voracious appetite, and obesity. Most Prader-Willi cases are associated with a specific abnormality on chromosome 15.

13. A 1997 consensus development conference convened by the U. S. Department of Health and Human Services Bureau of Maternal and Child Health made recommendations for basic laboratory testing in children which we will probably begin to follow. They include liver function tests to diagnose fatty liver, insulin levels to better assess glucose metabolism, and a fasting lipid profile to detect lipid disorders which are found among obese persons.

14. Other examples of autosomal recessive diseases are sickle cell disease, cystic fibrosis, and phenylketonuria (PKU). Diseases caused by an abnormal gene inherited from only one parent are known as autosomal dominant diseases; examples are familial hypercholesterolemia and neurofibromatosis. When a male child inherits a trait from the X chromosome of the mother, it is called X-linked inheritance; examples are color blindness, Duchenne's muscular dystrophy, and hemophilia.

Glossary

Adenosine triphosphate (ATP) A compound found in all living cells that stores the energy derived from food and transfers it for biological work.

Amino acid The basic building block of proteins.

Anorexia An eating disorder in which affected individuals (usually young females) have an intense fear of gaining weight or becoming fat (even though they may be underweight) and refuse to maintain a normal weight.

Apnea Absence of breathing.

Apoprotein The protein part of a protein complex. It can bind to lipids, including triglycerides, making it possible for the lipid to be dissolved in blood plasma.

Atherosclerosis A condition in which plaques containing cholesterol and fatty material are deposited inside arteries, where they can obstruct blood flow.

Atom The basic unit that characterizes an element.

Autonomic nervous system The part of the nervous system that controls involuntary functions, such as the activity of glands and heart muscle.

Binge eater A person who eats rapidly for at least two days a week until he or she feels uncomfortable and experiences guilt, remorse, or depression but does not use vomiting or purging to compensate for overeating.

Biostatistics The science of collecting, classifying, and analyzing biological facts or data.

Body mass The size or bulk of a person's body.

Body mass index The relationship of a person's weight and height.

Bulimia An eating disorder in which the affected person indulges in binge eating and then uses inappropriate methods, such as induced vomiting or purging with laxatives and diuretics, to compensate.

Carbohydrate A class of molecules that includes simple sugars, such as glucose, and complex substances made up of sugars, such as starch, glycogen, and cellulose.

Cardiomyopathy Disease of the heart muscle.

Celsius A temperature scale in which there are 100 equal divisions (degrees) between the freezing point (0 degrees) and the boiling point (100 degrees) of water at sea level.

Cholesterol The major sterol in the body. A sterol is a lipid found in most cell membranes which gives them structure; it also serves as a precursor to other products in the body, such as bile and certain hormones.

Cognition The act or process of knowing. The term includes perceiving, remembering, recognizing, conceiving, judging, sensing, reasoning, and imagining.

Cohort A group of people who experience a significant event, such as birth, at the same time.

Coronary arteries The blood vessels that supply the heart muscle.

Cortisol A hormone produced by the adrenal gland that helps regulate carbohydrate metabolism.

Cross-sectional study A "snapshot" examination of a population to determine how many people have a particular disease or condition at that point in time.

Demography The study of groups of people and their characteristics. An example is a study in which the people of Mississippi are classified according to their racial origin, whether they live in urban or rural settings, how many have automobiles, etc.

DNA (deoxyribonucleic acid) The molecule that genes are made of.

Diabetes mellitus A disease that results when blood glucose does not enter cells at a normal rate because of either a deficiency of insulin secretion or cellular resistance to insulin.

Dilation The act of stretching or the state of being stretched. "Dilation" must be differentiated from "hypertrophy," which is an increase in the bulk of an organ.

Electrolyte A compound that is able to conduct electricity when it is dissolved in water.

Electron The negatively charged subunit of an atom.

Element A substance composed of only one kind of atom.

Energy The capacity to do work.

Energy balance The state in which a person's energy intake and expenditure, over time, are equal.

Enzymes Highly specific catalysts that regulate the body's chemical reactions.

Excretion The process of removing undigested food and metabolic waste products from the body.

Fatty acid A component of fat molecules.

First law of thermodynamics A law in physics stating that in any physical or chemical change, the total amount of energy remains constant.

Food quotient (FQ) The ratio of volume of carbon dioxide produced to volume of oxygen consumed when a particular food is oxidized (burned).

Genotype A person's genetic makeup.

Gluconeogenesis The formation of glucose from molecules that are not themselves carbohydrates.

Glycogen The principal form of carbohydrate stored in the body.

Glycogenolysis The breaking down of glycogen to glucose.

Homeostasis The state of constancy of the body's internal environment.

Hypertension Abnormally high blood pressure.

Hypertrophy An increase in the bulk of an organ due to an increase in the size of the cells.

Hypoxemia Abnormally low oxygen content of arterial blood.

"Ideal" weight The weight that is appropriate for height.

Ion An atom or a group of atoms carrying an electrical charge, due to either gaining or losing one or more electrons.

Isotope One of two or more atoms having the same number of protons but a different number of neutrons, and hence, different weights.

Lipid A substance that is soluble in fat solvents (e.g., alcohol) but not in water.

Lipoprotein A compound made up of protein and lipid molecules.

Longitudinal study A study that takes place over time. For example, it might follow persons who are obese and those who are not and then determine the number in each group who eventually develop heart attacks or diabetes.

Macronutrients Nutrients required in large quantities, such as carbohydrates, proteins, and fats.

Mass, atomic Atomic weight.

Mass, body See **Body mass index**.

Molecule The smallest unit of a substance that retains the chemical properties of that substance.

Mutation Any permanent genetic change.

Neurotransmitter A chemical that is released by a nerve cell at its junction with another nerve cell, a muscle cell, or a gland, and which allows a nerve impulse to be transmitted.

Neutron An electrically neutral subunit of an atom, which, like a proton, contributes to its mass.

Obesity In this book, the condition in which body mass index (BMI) equals or exceeds the 95th reference standard percentile for age, sex, and race.

Obesity cardiomyopathy Disease of the heart muscle resulting from stress induced by obesity.

Overweight In this book, the condition in which body mass index (BMI) equals or exceeds the 85th reference standard percentile for age, sex, and race.

Percentile A value that divides a range of numbers (a "dataset") into two groups so that a given percentage lies below this value.

Phenotype Observable structural, biochemical, or molecular traits that follow from genetic and environmental influences.

Prepubertal Before puberty.

Prevalence The fraction (proportion) of a group having a disease or other characteristic at a particular point in time.

Protein A large molecule, made up of amino acids, which is important in cell structure and which forms enzymes, antibodies, and hormones.

Proton An electrically positive subunit of an atom, which, like a neutron, contributes to its mass.

Puberty The stage of onset of sexual maturity.

Receptor A molecular structure on or in a cell that binds specifically with a factor such as a hormone or a neurotransmitter, causing a cellular effect.

Respiratory quotient (RQ) The ratio of the volume of carbon dioxide released to the volume of oxygen consumed per unit time; a measure of metabolic activity.

Secretion The release of chemical substances made by a cell or a gland.

Starch A carbohydrate molecule consisting of a long chain of repeating units of glucose.

Sugar Any one of a class of sweet, water soluble, crystalline carbohydrates, such as glucose, fructose, and lactose.

Triglyceride (triacylglycerol) A compound consisting of three fatty acid molecules bound to one glycerol molecule.

Ventricles (heart) The two pumping chambers of the heart. The right ventricle pumps blood to the lung, and the left ventricle pumps it to the rest of the body.

Work The transfer of force from one body or system to another.

References

Abenhaim, L., Y. Moride, F. Brenot, et al. 1996. Appetite-suppressant drugs and the risk of primary pulmonary hypertension. *New England Journal of Medicine* 335: 609–16.

Acheson, K., J-P Flatt, and E. Jequier. 1982. Glycogen synthesis vs. lipogenesis after a 500-gram carbohydrate meal in man. *Metabolism* 31: 1234–40.

Alpert, M. A., and M. W. Hashimi. 1993. Obesity and the heart. *American Journal of the Medical Sciences* 306 (2): 117–23.

Anonymous. 1996. Long-term pharmacotherapy in the management of obesity. National Task Force on the Prevention and Treatment of Obesity. *Journal of the American Medical Association* 276 (23): 1907–15.

Ballard-Barbash, R., and C. A. Swanson. 1996. Body weight: Estimation of risk for breast and endometrial cancers. *American Journal of Clinical Nutrition* 63 (supplement): 437S–41S.

Bandini, L. G., D. A. Schoeller, H. Cyr, et al. 1990. Validity of reported energy intake in obese and non-obese adolescents. *American Journal of Clinical Nutrition* 52: 421–25.

Bao, W., S. R. Srinivasan, R. Valdez, et al. 1997. Longitudinal changes in cardiovascular risk from childhood to young adulthood in offspring of parents with coronary artery disease. The Bogalusa Heart Study. *Journal of the American Medical Association* 278: 1749–54.

Bistrian, B. 1978. Clinical use of a protein-sparing modified fast. *Journal of the American Medical Association* 240 (21): 2299–2302.

Boeck, M., K. Lubin, I. Loy, et al. 1993. Initial experience with long-term inpatient treatment of morbidly obese children in a rehabilitation facility. *Annals of the New York Academy of Sciences* 699: 257–59.

Bogardus, C., S. Lillioja, and E. Ravussin. 1986. Familial dependence of the resting metabolic rate. *New England Journal of Medicine* 315: 96–100.

Borjeson, M. 1976. The aetiology of obesity in children: A study of 101 twin pairs. *Acta Paediatrica Scandinavica* 65: 279–87.

Borrud, L. 1997. Eating out in America: Impact on food choices and nutrient profiles. http://www.barc.usda.gov.../foodsurvey/eatout95.htm

Bouchard, C., A. Tremblay, A. Nadeau, et al. 1989. Genetic effect in resting and exercise metabolic rates. *Metabolism* 38 (4): 364–70.

Bouchard, C., A. Tremblay, J-P Després, et al. 1990. The response to long-term overfeeding in identical twins. *New England Journal of Medicine* 322: 1477–82.

Bouchard, C., and L. Pèrusse. 1993. Genetics of obesity. *Annual Reviews of Nutrition* 13: 337–54.

Bouchard, C., A. Tremblay, J-P Després, et al. 1994. The response to exercise with constant energy intake in identical twins. *Obesity Research* 59: 975–79.

Bougnères, P., C. Le Stunff, C. Pecqueur, et al. 1997. In vivo resistance of lipolysis to epinephrine: A new feature of childhood onset obesity. *Journal of Clinical Investigation* 99 (11): 2568–73.

Bray, G. A. 1985. Complications of obesity. *Annals of Internal Medicine* 103 (6 part 2): 1052–62.

Campfield, L. A., F. J. Smith, Y. Guisez, et al. 1995. Recombinant mouse ob protein: Evidence for a peripheral signal linking adiposity and central neural networks. *Science* 269: 546–49.

Centers for Disease Control and Prevention. 1991. Participation of high school students in school physical education—United States, 1990. *Morbidity and Mortality Weekly Report* 40: 607–15.

———. 1992. Vigorous physical activity among high school students—United States, 1990. *Morbidity and Mortality Weekly Report* 41: 33–35.

———. 1996. State-specific prevalence of participation in physical activity. Behavioral Risk Factor Surveillance System. *Morbidity and Mortality Weekly Report* 45: 673–75.

———. 1996. Guidelines for school health programs to promote lifelong healthy eating. *Morbidity and Mortality Weekly Report* 45 (RR-9): 1–37.

———. 1997. Update: Prevalence of overweight among children, adolescents, and adults—United States, 1988–94. *Morbidity and Mortality Weekly Report* 46: 199–202.

Clèment, K., C. Vaisse, B. S. J. Manning, et al. 1995. Genetic variation in the ß₃-adrenergic receptor and an increased capacity to gain weight in patients with morbid obesity. *New England Journal of Medicine* 333: 352–54.

Coleman, D. L. 1973. Effects of parabiosis of obese with diabetes and normal mice. *Diabetologia* 9: 294–98.

Connolly, H. M., J. L. Crary, M. D. McGoon, et al. 1997. Valvular heart disease associated with fenfluramine-phentermine. *New England Journal of Medicine* 337: 581–88.

Davies, P. S. W., J. M. E. Day, and A. Lucas. 1991. Energy expenditure in early infancy and later body fatness. *International Journal of Obesity* 15: 727–31.

Dietz, W. H. 1994. Critical periods in childhood for the development of obesity. *American Journal of Clinical Nutrition* 59: 955–59.

Dietz, W. H., and T. N. Robinson. 1993. Assessment and treatment of childhood obesity. *Pediatrics in Review* 14 (9): 337–43.

Drewnowski, A., and C. L. Rock. 1995. The influence of genetic taste markers on food acceptance. *American Journal of Clinical Nutrition* 62 (3): 506–11.

Eckel, R. H., and R. M. Krauss. 1998. American Heart Association call to action: Obesity as a major risk factor for coronary artery disease. AHA Nutrition Committee (news) *Circulation* 97 (21): 2099–2100.

Epstein, L. H., and S. Squires. 1988. *The stoplight diet for children: An eight-week program for parents and children*. Boston: Little, Brown and Company.

Epstein, L. H., A. Valoski, R. R. Wing, et al. 1990. Ten-year follow-up of behavioral, family-based treatment for obese children. *Journal of the American Medical Association* 264: 2519–23.

Erickson, J. C., K. E. Klegg, and P. D. Palmiter. 1996. Sensitivity to leptin and susceptibility to seizures of mice lacking neuropeptide Y. *Nature* 381: 415–18.

Flatt, J. P. 1993. Dietary fat, carbohydrate balance, and weight maintenance. *Annals of the New York Academy of Sciences* 683: 122–40.

———. 1995. Use and storage of carbohydrate and fat. *American Journal of Clinical Nutrition* 61 (supplement): 952S–59S.

Foster, G. D., T. A. Wadden, and R. A. Vogt. 1997. Resting energy expenditure in obese African American and Caucasian women. *Obesity Research* 5 (1): 1–8.

Garn, S. M., and M. LaVelle. 1985. Two-decade follow-up of fatness in early childhood. *American Journal of Diseases of Children* 139: 181–85.

Garrow, J. S. 1988. Aetiology of obesity in man. Chap. 6 in *Obesity and related diseases*. Edinburgh: Churchill Livingstone.

Gortmaker, S. L., A. Must, A. M. Sobol, et al. 1996. Television viewing as a cause of increasing obesity among children in the United States, 1986–1990. *Archives of Pediatric and Adolescent Medicine* 150: 356–62.

Guo, S., A. F. Roche, and L. Houtkooper. 1989. Fat-free mass in children and young adults predicted from bioelectric impedance and anthropometric variables. *American Journal of Clinical Nutrition* 50: 435–43.

Guo, S. S., A. F. Roche, W. C. Chumlea, et al. 1994. The predictive value of childhood body mass index values for overweight at age 35y. *American Journal of Clinical Nutrition* 59: 810–19.

Guyton, A. C. 1981. *Textbook of medical physiology*. 6th ed. Philadelphia: W. B. Saunders Co.

Halaas, J., K. S. Gajiwala, M. Maffei, et al. 1995. Weight-reducing effects of the plasma protein encoded by the *obese* gene. *Science* 269: 543–46.

Hamann, A., and S. Matthaie. 1996. Regulation of energy balance by leptin. *Experimental and Clinical Endocrinology and Diabetes* 104: 293–300.

Hammer, L. D. 1992. The development of eating behavior in childhood. *Pediatric Clinics of North America* 39: 379–94.

Heath, G. W., M. Pratt, and C. W. Warren. 1994. Physical activity patterns in American high school students. Results from the 1990 Youth Risk Behavior Survey. *Archives of Pediatric and Adolescent Medicine* 148: 1131–36.

Hervey, G. R. 1959. The effects of lesions in the hypothalamus in parabiotic rats. *Journal of Physiology* 145: 336–52.

Higgins, M., W. Kannel, R. Garrison, et al. 1987. Hazards of obesity: The Framingham experience. *Acta Medica Scandinavica* 723 (supplement): 23–36.

Hill, J. O., M. J. Pagliassotti, and J. C. Peters. 1994. Nongenetic determinants of obesity and body fat topography. Chap. 3 in *The Genetics of Obesity*, ed. C. Bouchard. Boca Raton, FL: CRC Press.

Horm, J., and K. Anderson. 1993. Who in America is trying to lose weight? *Annals of Internal Medicine* 119 (7): 672–76.

Huang, Z., S. E. Hankinson, G. A. Colditz, et al. 1997. Dual effects of weight and weight gain on breast cancer risk. *Journal of the American Medical Association* 278 (17): 1407–11.

Johnson, S. L., and L. L. Birch. 1994. Parents' and children's adiposity and eating style. *Pediatrics* 94: 653–61.

Kaplan, A. S., B. S. Zemil, and V. A. Stallings. 1996. Differences in resting energy expenditure in prepubertal black children and white children. *Journal of Pediatrics* 129: 643–47.

Katch, F., E. D. Michael, and S. M. Horvath. 1967. Estimation of body volume by underwater weighing: Description of a simple method. *Journal of Applied Physiology* 23 (5): 811–13.

Kennedy, G. C. 1953. The role of depot fat in the hypothalamic control of food intake in the rat. *Proceedings of the Royal Society of London (Biology)* 140: 578–92.

Kennedy, E., and J. Goldberg. 1995. What are American children eating? Implications for public policy. *Nutrition Reviews* 53 (5): III–26.

Kimm, S. Y. S., E. Obarzanek, B. A. Barton, et al. 1996. Race, socioeconomic status, and obesity in 9- and 10-year-old girls: The NHLBI Growth and Health Study. *Annals of Epidemiology* 6: 266–75.

Kral, J. G. 1992. Overview of surgical techniques for treating obesity. *American Journal of Clinical Nutrition* 55 (supplement): 552S–55S.

Kuczmarski, R. J., K. M. Flegal, S. M. Campbell, et al. 1994. Increasing prevalence of overweight among U.S. adults. The National Health and Nutrition Examination Surveys, 1960 to 1991. *Journal of the American Medical Association* 272: 205–11.

Kumanyika, S. 1987. Obesity in black women. *Epidemiologic Reviews* 9: 31–50.

Kumanyika, S., J. F. Wilson, and M. Guilford-Davenport. 1993. Weight-related attitudes and behaviors of black women. *Journal of the American Dietetic Association* 93: 416–22.

Leibel, R. L., M. Rosenbaum, and J. Hirsch. 1995. Changes in energy expenditure resulting from altered body weight. *New England Journal of Medicine* 332: 621–28.

Lew, E. A. 1985. Mortality and weight: Insured lives and the American Cancer Society Studies. *Annals of Internal Medicine* 103 (6 part 2): 1024–29.

Luepker, R. V., C. L. Perry, S. M. McKinlay, et al. 1996. Outcomes of a field trial to improve children's dietary patterns and physical activity. The Child and Adolescent Trial for Cardiovascular Health (CATCH). *Journal of the American Medical Association* 275: 768–76.

Maffei, M., J. Halaas, E. Ravussin, et al. 1995. Leptin levels in human and rodent: Measurement of plasma leptin and *ob* RNA in obese and weight-reduced subjects. *Nature Medicine* 1: 1155–58.

Massachusetts Medical Society Committee on Nutrition. 1989. Fast food fare: Consumer guidelines. *New England Journal of Medicine* 321 (11): 752–56.

McCann, U. D., L. S. Seiden, L. J. Rubin, et al. 1997. Brain serotonin neurotoxicity and primary pulmonary hypertension from fenfluramine and dexfenfluramine. A systematic review of the evidence. *Journal of the American Medical Association* 278: 666–72.

McNutt, S. W., Y. Hu, G. B. Schreiber, et al. 1997. A longitudinal study of the dietary practices of black and white girls 9 and 10 years old at enrollment: The NHLBI Growth and Health Study. *Journal of Adolescent Health* 20: 27–37.

Melnyk, M. G., and E. Weinstein. 1994. Preventing obesity in black women by targeting adolescents: A literature review. *Journal of the American Dietetic Association* 94: 536–40.

Moore, L. L., D. A. Lombardi, M. J. White, et al. 1991. Influence of parents' physical activity levels on activity levels of young children. *Journal of Pediatrics* 118: 215–19.

Morrison, J. A., M. P. Alfaro, P. Khoury, et al. 1996. Determinants of resting energy expenditure in young black girls and young white girls. *Journal of Pediatrics* 129: 637–42.

Muñoz, K. A., S. M. Krebs-Smith, R. Ballard-Barbash, et al. 1997. Food intakes of U. S. children and adolescents compared with recommendations. *Pediatrics* 100 (3): 323–29.

National Institute of Diabetes and Digestive and Kidney Diseases (NIDDK) Home Page. 1997. Diabetes Statistics. http://www.niddk. nih.gov/DiabetesStatistics/DiabetesStatistics.html.

———. 1997. Statistics related to overweight and obesity. http://www.niddk.nih.gov/obstats/obstats.htm.

National Institutes of Health Consensus Conference Statement. 1985. Health implications of obesity. *Annals of Internal Medicine* 103 (6 part 2): 1073–77.

National Institutes of Health Technology Assessment Conference Panel. 1992. Methods for voluntary weight loss and control. *Annals of Internal Medicine* 116: 942–49.

National Institutes of Health Consensus Statement. 1995. Physical Activity and Cardiovascular Health. 13: 1–33.

National Task Force on the Prevention and Treatment of Obesity. 1993. Very low-calorie diets. *Journal of the American Medical Association* 270 (8): 967–74.

Ogden, C. L., R. P. Troiano, R. R. Briefel, et al. 1997. Prevalence of overweight among preschool children in the United States, 1971 through 1994. *Pediatrics* 99 (4). URL:http://www.pediatrics.lorg/dgi/content/full/99/4/e1.

Oliveria, S. A., R. C. Ellison, L. L. Moore, et al. 1992. Parent-child relationships in nutrient intake: The Framingham Children's Study. *American Journal of Clinical Nutrition* 56 (3): 593–98.

Pate, R. R., M. Dowda, and J. G. Ross. 1990. Associations between physical activity and physical fitness in American children. *American Journal of Diseases of Children* 144: 1123–29.

Pate, R. R., M. Pratt, S. N. Blair, et al. 1995. Physical activity and public health: A recommendation from the Centers for Disease Control and Prevention and the American College of Sports Medicine. *Journal of the American Medical Association* 273: 402–7.

Perri, M. G., A. M. Nezu, and B. J. Viegener. 1992. *Improving the long-term management of obesity: Theory, research, and clinical guidelines.* New York: John Wiley and Sons.

Pica, R. 1995. *Experiences in movement with music, activities, and theory.* Albany: Delmar Publishers Inc.

Pinhas-Hamiel, O., L. M. Dolan, S. R. Daniels, et al. 1996. Increased incidence of non-insulin-dependent diabetes mellitus among adolescents. *Journal of Pediatrics* 128: 608–15.

Pi-Sunyer, F. X. 1991. Health implications of obesity. *American Journal of Clinical Nutrition* 53 (supplement): 1595S–1603S.

Prentice, A. M., A. E. Black, W. A. Coward, et al. 1986. High levels of energy expenditure in obese women. *British Medical Journal* 292: 983–87.

Prochaska, J. O., C. C. DiClemente, and J. C. Norcross. 1992. In search of how people change: Applications to addictive behaviors. *American Psychologist* 47: 1102–14.

Ravussin, E., S. Lillioja, W. C. Knowler, et al. 1988. Reduced rate of energy expenditure as a risk factor for body-weight gain. *New England Journal of Medicine* 318: 467–72.

Roberts, S. B., J. Savage, W. A. Coward, et al. 1988. Energy expenditure and intake in infants born to lean and overweight mothers. *New England Journal of Medicine* 318: 461–66.

Ross, J. G., and R. R. Pate. 1987. The National Children and Youth Fitness Study III. A summary of findings. *Journal of Physical Education, Recreation, and Dance* (November–December).

Schreiber, G. B., M. Robins, R. Striegel-Moore, et al. 1996. Weight modification efforts reported by black and white preadolescent girls: National Heart, Lung, and Blood Institute Growth and Health Study. *Pediatrics* 98 (1): 63–70.

Schwartz, M. W., and R. J. Seeley. 1997. The new biology of body weight regulation. *Journal of the American Dietetic Association* 97 (1): 54–58.

Serdula, M. K., M. E. Collins, D. F. Williamson, et al. 1993. Weight control practices of U.S. adolescents and adults. *Annals of Internal Medicine* 119: 667–71.

Serdula, M. K., D. Ivery, R. J. Coates, et al. 1993. Do obese children become obese adults? A review of the literature. *Preventive Medicine* 22: 167–77.

Shike, M. 1996. Body weight and colon cancer. *American Journal of Clinical Nutrition* 63 (supplement): 4425–45.

Siri, W. E. 1956. The gross composition of the body. *Advances in Biology, Medicine, and Physics* 4: 239–80.

Smith, J. C., W. H. Sorey, D. Quebedeau, et al. 1997. Use of body mass index to monitor treatment of obese adolescents. *Journal of Adolescent Health* 20: 466–69.

Smith, J. C., C. Field, D. S. Braden, et al. 1999. Coexisting health problems in obese children and adolescents that might require special treatment considerations. *Clinical Pediatrics* (in press).

Stanley, B. G., S. E. Kyrkouli, S. Lampert, et al. 1986. Neuropeptide Y chronically injected into the hypothalamus: A powerful neurochemical inducer of hyperphagia and obesity. *Peptides* 7: 1189–92.

Stunkard, A. J., T. I. A. Sørensen, C. Hanis, et al. 1986. An adoption study of human obesity. *New England Journal of Medicine* 314: 193–98.

Stunkard, A. J., T. T. Foch, and Z. Hrubec. 1986. A twin study of human obesity. *Journal of the American Medical Association* 256: 51–54.

Stunkard, A. J., J. R. Harris, N. L. Pedersen, et al. 1990. The body-mass index of twins who have been reared apart. *New England Journal of Medicine* 322: 1483–87.

Swinburn, B., and E. Ravussin. 1993. Energy balance or fat balance? *American Journal of Clinical Nutrition* 57 (supplement): 766S–71S.

Tartaglia, L. A., M. Dembski, X. Weng, et al. 1995. Identification and expression cloning of a leptin receptor, OB-R. *Cell* 83: 1263–71.

Troiano, R. P., K. M. Flegal, R. J. Kuczmarski, et al. 1995. Overweight prevalence and trends for children and adolescents. The National Health and Nutrition Examination Surveys, 1963 to 1991. *Archives of Pediatric and Adolescent Medicine* 149: 1085–91.

United States Department of Agriculture Web Site. 1995. Nutrition and your health: Dietary guidelines for Americans. Fourth Edition. http://www.usda.gov/fcs/library/0102-1.txt.

United States Department of Health and Human Services. 1991. Healthy People 2000: National health promotion and disease prevention objectives. DHHS Publication No. (PHS) 91-50212, U. S. Government Printing Office, Washington DC.

———. 1996. Physical activity and health: A report of the surgeon general. Atlanta, GA: U.S. Department of Health and Human Services, Centers for Disease Control and Prevention, National Center for Chronic Disease Prevention and Health Promotion.

Weinsier, R. L., K. M. Nelson, D. D. Hensrud, et al. 1995. Metabolic predictors of obesity. Contribution of resting energy expenditure, thermic effect of food, and fuel utilization to four-year weight gain of post-obese and never-obese women. *Journal of Clinical Investigation* 95: 980–85.

Whitaker, R. C., J. A. Wright, M. S. Pepe, et al. 1997. Predicting obesity in young adulthood from childhood and parental obesity. *New England Journal of Medicine* 337: 869–73.

Wolf, A. M., and G. A. Colditz. 1994. The costs of obesity: The U.S. perspective. *Pharmacoeconomics* 5: 34–37.

Zhang, Y., R. Proenca, M. Maffel, et al. 1994. Positional cloning of the mouse *obese* gene and its human homologue. *Nature* 372: 425–32.

Index

Note: (t) refers to a table; (f) refers to a figure.